THE
HEALING
POWER
OF
HADO

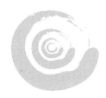

THE
HEALING
POWER
OF
HADO

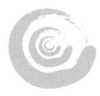

TOYOKO MATSUZAKI
WITH NATSUMI BLACKWELL

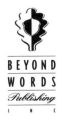

BEYOND
WORDS
Publishing
I   N   C

Beyond Words Publishing, Inc.
20827 N.W. Cornell Road, Suite 500
Hillsboro, Oregon 97124-9808
503-531-8700

Editor: Julie Steigerwaldt
Managing editor: Sarabeth Blakey
Proofreader: Jade Chan
Design: Jerry Soga
Composition: William H. Brunson Typography Services

Printed in the United States of America
Distributed to the book trade by Publishers Group West

Library of Congress Cataloging-in-Publication Data

Matsuzaki, Toyoko.
    The healing power of hado / Toyoko Matsuzaki with
Natsumi Blackwell.
        p. cm.
    1. Touch—Therapeutic use.   2. Vital force—Therapeutic use.
3. Imposition of hands—Therapeutic use.   4. Aura.   5. Traditional
medicine—Japan.   I. Blackwell, Natsumi.   II. Title.

RZ999.M35   2004
615.8'22—dc22

                                                          2004029973

Disclaimer:
The information offered in this book is for educational purposes only. It is not intended as a replacement for the expertise of a qualified health-care provider. Neither the publisher nor the authors accept responsibility for any effects that may arise from the correct or incorrect use of information in this book.

The corporate mission of Beyond Words Publishing, Inc.:
    Inspire to Integrity

To Takaori, my only child,
who inspired me to write this book

CONTENTS

Acknowledgments

My deepest gratitude goes to Cynthia Black at Beyond Words Publishing, who trusted in me and guided me though the publishing process. I can never thank her enough. It has been great working with her.

I also thank Julie Steigerwaldt, who patiently edited the manuscript. Her literary skills made the book more focused and useful.

Thanks also to Richard Cohn at Beyond Words, and Rosalyn Voget Neumann for her editorial input.

I also appreciate the many others who connected me to the right people to publish this book. Thank you all.

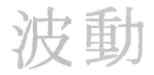

Introduction

What exactly is *hado*? Have you ever entered a room full of people and sensed the mood, without anyone saying a word? Or felt calm and lighter after receiving a warm hug from a friend when your spirits were down? If so, you've experienced the effects of hado firsthand. Hado is the life force found in everything. You can harness this power to enrich your own life and improve the world around you.

In English, hado translates as "wave motion" or "vibration." The word has existed in Japanese for centuries, but within the past few decades it has begun to be used in the context of philosophy, science, and quantum physics. (You may be familiar with the work of Dr. Masaru Emoto, a Japanese scientist who studies the remarkable effects of hado on water crystals.) Recently the definition of hado has expanded into the spiritual realm to express the healing properties and transformative power of this life-force energy.

Once you begin to study hado, the possibilities are endless. Beginners can receive messages from the hado released by other people, objects, and environments. At a more advanced level, practitioners of hado can change the essences of physical materials. (For example, they can make jewelry sparkle or change the taste of water.) Those who practice hado at the master level can heal physical ailments of their own and of others (hands-on or remotely), discover their clairvoyant abilities, and even receive messages from departed loved ones.

As you read this book, I will be your guide as you become familiar with the healing power of hado. We'll begin with an introduction to the concept of hado, then move on to examples from my experience and those of my clients, and an explanation of how to tap into your own power. At the end of the book you'll find lessons and tips for continued practice.

I have been a hado master for twenty-two years, helping clients such as business professionals, artists, musicians, physicians, lawyers, and *kabuki* (traditional Japanese theater) actors, among many others. I believe I was born with exceptional hado power, although I did not start to realize its full potential and study it until I was thirty-eight years old. Because using hado comes as naturally to me as breathing, it is difficult to explicitly illustrate how I do it. How do you teach another how to pray? So I offer my experience and tools to help you discover your own abilities within yourself. Though I try to be as specific and as clear as possible, you will find that your own way is unique. I encourage you to be creative, test your limits, and explore the paths on which the practice of hado takes you.

As a professional hado master, I am kept very busy with requests for healing from people all over Japan and Taiwan, and international demand for my work is growing. Because I am only human, I cannot reach everyone who seeks my help. My hope is that this book will be a stand-in for my personal services so that people can use hado power when I cannot be there for them physically. You can also look at my picture or visualize me to be connected to my hado. It doesn't matter if I'm on the opposite side of the globe; my hado will come through to you to benefit you and your loved ones.

To help you understand how I came to be a hado master, I would like to tell you a little about my life. I grew up in Osaka, Japan, during the aftermath of World War II. Japan was still under U.S. occupation, and it was an era of chaos. From early on I felt that I possessed a kind of clairvoyant power. Of course I never imagined that I would be a hado master or write a book about hado, but I always had vivid pictures in my mind, such as driving a car by myself as an adult and visiting many places. People used to laugh at my wild imagination, because Japanese people were still very poor at that time, and only millionaires owned their own cars. I also had a strong sense that I would be alone.

When I was fifteen, I entered a choral contest and felt sure that I would win first prize. Again, people laughed at my wild imagination, but I got the first prize as I had predicted. The following year, everybody expected me to win again, but I knew that it was not going to happen. Again, I was correct.

As a teenager, I had strange dreams, but they were more than dreams; they felt like visions located between the real world and the dream world. In one vision, a beautiful angel with plumage stepped from a carriage that had descended from heaven and extended her hands to me. In awe, I touched her hand, hoping that she would take me to heaven; however, she just gave me a gentle smile and held my hand. The dream was so vivid, and even now I can still clearly remember everything in it, including the angel's face and her beautiful plumage. (At that time I attended a high school called Plumage Private Academy.) When I had this dream the first time, I was young and didn't think much about its meaning. But after having the same dream three times, I started to feel that it was a sign. I have come to believe that the angel in my dream was passing her hado power on to me by touching my hands.

Shortly after having these dreams, I decided to study vocal music seriously. At the time, there was an opera singer who had a beautiful voice, and I wanted to be like her. I think my dreams about the angel also gave me the extra boost in self-confidence that I needed to study vocal music. While applying to one of the most prestigious music colleges in Tokyo, I had a strong feeling that I would pass the entrance examination with a high score. I called my parents and said in a loud voice, "I think I will make the top score!" I still remember that one of the teachers overheard me. How young and sassy I must have sounded! But just as I had imagined, I passed the examination with the top score.

After graduating from college, I totally devoted myself to music as a professional singer. I became a member of one of the largest opera companies in Japan and appeared on many stages. I really loved singing and lived my life to the fullest. I realize now that this part of my background was crucial to the hado power I would discover later in my life. Hado and sound are very similar because both consist of unseen wave motion, or vibrations, and you have to nurture your sensitivity to wave motion to be a singer or a hado master. I also studied how to use my body to produce good sound; for example, I learned which part of the body to aim at when singing in front of an audience. I learned how to breathe, to circulate the oxygen in my body from head to toe. (Not only did this help my singing but it also improved my posture and contributed to my good health.) This training gave me a firm foundation when I later began to develop my hado power.

As I grew older, my clairvoyant inklings continued to be a force in my life. Before giving birth to my son, Takaori, I went for a regular checkup at a clinic where my family had connections. I felt uneasy about the clinic and checked my medical chart in private. To my surprise, it listed the wrong blood type for me. I decided to go to another hospital without consulting anyone. When I started having contractions, I asked a nurse if this hospital was capable of performing C-sections. The nurse said yes.

My labor was terribly long and painful. I told a nurse that I wanted to give up, but she said that I couldn't stop until I delivered my baby. As labor progressed to forty-eight hours, the heartbeat of my unborn baby became weak. The doctors finally decided to do a C-section, and I was finally able to hold my son. It was fortunate that I had changed hospitals, for the doctors at the other clinic couldn't perform C-sections, and even if they could have, they might have given me the wrong blood type.

After my son was born, the nurse said, "You asked me about a C-section earlier. You must have felt something at that time." I strongly feel that both my son and I were protected by guardian angels to have had such a successful outcome.

When I was thirty-eight, my mother had a stroke, and her body became partially paralyzed. To alleviate her pain, I would massage her body. While I was doing this, something strong welled up from deep within my soul, and I knew that something miraculous was happening. I continued to rub my mother's arms and legs, praying for her recovery. I was sending her my own hado power without even realizing it. Strangely enough, she told me that her body became lighter and lighter and warmer and warmer after I gave her massages. After some time, her paralysis was gone. I had sent my healing energy—my hado power—and healed her paralysis without instruction from anyone. The doctor told me that it was a true miracle that she recovered fully from her paralysis. In her follow-up visits, the doctors couldn't find any evidence of the paralysis at all.

After my mother's miraculous recovery, I tried to understand and practice this new healing ability. I made many mistakes while I was developing the power—mistakes that I learned much from. My family was very generous in letting me practice hado healing on their bodies, and I am grateful to them. One day I sent hado power into a relative's sore arm. I must have sent too much because she started to complain that her arm felt heavy and uncomfortable. I didn't know how to fix it, and she decided to take a bath. Then I heard her yell from the bathroom, "Something came out of my elbow!" She had seen something like a Ping-Pong ball moving around inside her arm, and then it felt like it left her body. I examined her arm; everything was normal, but she said that it no longer felt heavy. Perhaps, I thought, the hado energy had left her body through that joint. This is how I learned that I have to make "exits," by applying pressure to an area I'm working on whenever I send hado power directly into the body. The way hado exits the body is different in each individual, and it varies with body build; for example, some people experience shaking in the arms and legs. Without making exits for the hado, the person being worked on may experience neck, shoulder, or leg cramps, and may have difficulty walking.

Through word of mouth, people heard of my mother's miraculous recovery and began to visit me. As more family members and friends asked me for help, I began to practice hado power more deeply, literally as on-the-job training. The more I used my hado power, the more I started to get readings from clients without even knowing them. This was my clairvoyant power kicking in. Clairvoyant power doesn't always come with hado power, but for some people it does. Before I knew it, people who needed help with relationships started to knock on my door, too. So I studied clairvoyant power as well through this on-the-job training.

Later, I developed new applications of hado power, such as changing the essences of materials and communicating with the dead.

I believe that I inherited my hado power from my parents (but someone who doesn't inherit the power can develop it through training, sometimes to a greater degree than one whose ability was passed down through blood). My family's history gives me reason to believe that my hado power was inherited. My mother's family ran a cotton spinning factory in Osaka. One night when my mother was young, she felt ill at ease about one of the warehouses. She couldn't sleep, so she went to the factory in the middle of the night to put a fire extinguisher at the door of the warehouse. The next day, a fire broke out at the warehouse, but thanks to the fire extinguisher my mother had left, the damage was minimal. On another occasion, she had an uneasy feeling and looked inside the factory from a hole in the wall. She saw a factory manager put some textiles into his pockets. When she told her father what she had seen, her father scolded her and said that she should not call anyone a thief. So she ran to the factory manager, stopped him at the gate, and asked one of the employees to check his pockets. The employee discovered that the manager had taken many textiles.

My late son, Takaori, had stronger hado power than I have. Without learning from him, I couldn't have so profoundly understood hado power and the law of nature. When Takaori was young, he loved to accompany his grandfather to play *pachinko* (Japanese pinball). Before going out, my son would often tell me that they didn't need dinner because they were going to eat out. At the pachinko place, my son would point to a particular machine and whisper to his grandfather, "Grandpa, I think you can hit the jackpot at that pachinko machine there!" My father always followed his advice because my son was always right. After making some cash, they would have dinner at Takaori's favorite steak restaurant near my house. Clairvoyant power does not usually work for gambling, but I suppose it did for Takaori because he was so young and innocent and only wanted to eat his favorite food with his grandfather.

Takaori loved cars and dreamed of being a professional racer one day, so he decided to attend vocational school to be a car mechanic. He chose the most prestigious and strictest school in Japan; students who failed even one term examination would have to leave the school. Before an examination, Takaori used to ask me to send my hado power to him. One time he reported to me that he couldn't remember a formula during the exam; then he thought about me and asked for my help. Suddenly, he had a vision of the formula as if it were on a TV screen, and he passed that test. At the time I thought he was exaggerating just to make me happy, but a while later, one of my vocal students asked me to send her my hado power before an examination. She, too, reported that the answer to a difficult question appeared as if on a TV screen when she thought about me for help. I was so excited after hearing about these episodes that I sent a little too much hado into my son at his next examination. He called me and complained that his body felt as if it were floating above the chair and he had a hard time concentrating.

My son also had exceptional clairvoyant power. One day I lost my purse. As I was about to call the credit card company to report that my card was missing, my son said, "Mother, you don't have to do that. I know where it is. On the way back home, you stopped by the parking lot of a restaurant some ten miles away from home, right? Your purse is still there."

We drove back to the restaurant together, and as soon as I parked the car, my son ran out to a small stream next to the parking lot and returned with my purse. He told me that he had had a vision of it near the stream.

When Takaori was twenty-six years old I awoke one night to the kind of phone call every parent fears. It was my son, calling to tell me he had been in an accident. He said, "Please don't worry about me. I am OK. I am safe now. I was riding a motorcycle home, and an SUV crashed into me."

I rushed to the hospital where he was being treated. The police told me that the vehicle had ignored the light and hit him. It was a miracle that my son wasn't hurt. According to him, when he was hit by the vehicle, he was thrown into the air, but somebody—we both knew that it was his favorite late grandfather—held him perfectly away from harm. I thanked my father for protecting my son from danger. It was then that I learned that the spirits of the departed stay with loved ones to protect them whenever they can.

This incident was only a sign of a real tragedy to come. Exactly one year after the motorcycle accident, I washed and set my hair before going to bed because I felt that I should be prepared for something that was coming. I received another call in the middle of the night. This time, it was the police; my son had been killed in a car accident. The next morning, I received an auto racing magazine with an article about my son, reporting on his debut in the coming month as a professional racer at the International Suzuka Circuit.

It is impossible to imagine the agony of a mother who has lost her only child. After the accident, I felt like I was going mad with grief, and I suffered for so long. I thought, "If only it had been me instead of him. How I am going to live without him?" I felt a strong urge to know about my son's last moments, so I went to the hospital to visit his friend, who had been driving the car and had survived with a broken leg. He told me about something unusual that had happened a few nights earlier. He couldn't sleep, so he left his hospital room to watch TV in the lobby. Suddenly the TV lost its reception and he felt a chill—the presence of my son. He immediately understood that my son had come to see if he was OK, since Takaori had such a big heart. My son's friend couldn't stop crying, because he was very touched; not only had my son forgiven him, but Takaori had been worried about his friend and the guilt he was feeling over the accident. This young man had never felt the presence of a departed person before but now totally believed in life after death.

I burst into tears upon hearing this story. It was not easy to do, but I firmly decided that I would forgive this person as Takaori had done, and treat him as if he were my son. I believe that it was Takaori's wish. I felt his presence, too; he told me that I was doing the right thing.

For years after Takaori's death I felt empty, like I would never smile or feel happy again. Then one night my son appeared to me in a dream. He must have been worried about me because I had been devastated over the loss of him for such a long time. He said, "Mother, please don't worry about me. I am OK. Work hard on your hado healing and help more people who are in pain. I really loved your smile when you were helping people in need."

When I woke up, I saw a small shaft of light and the words *Kokoro no Orion* (Weaving the Sound of Heart) in my mind. I used my clairvoyant power with hado and had a vision of a booklet with that title. As a result of that vision, I wrote and published a booklet about how I solved the problems of my clients, such as healing the sick and delivering messages from the dead, with my hado power. To my surprise, many copies of the booklet were distributed in a short period of time without any advertising. I received many calls from readers, and I traveled all across Japan to help them solve their problems. I saw so many miracles, and I know this was a precious gift from my son.

After this dream, I felt that it was time to live my life again. It had been my son's time to go and his fate. It was not easy to accept the tragedy, but I knew that he had lived his life to the fullest. I had to move on. Luckily I had—and still have—a job to do as a hado master and many people to help.

The real gift from my son is being able to reach people all over the world and to teach them about hado and the laws of nature. When I began writing the book you hold in your hands, I started to feel a strange pain in my stomach and I wondered why; then I realized that the pain was very similar to the contractions I felt when I gave birth to Takaori. I was giving birth again—this time to my son's book, my son's gift. I strongly felt that the time was right to begin working on this expanded book about hado. I sensed my son's spirit right next to me, and he said, "Yes, Mother, the time has come. Start writing."

I
Hado Power

波動

What Is Hado?

In ancient Chinese medicine and philosophy, everything releases energy, or *qi*. Recently in Japan, people in the spiritual community have started to use the word hado to express a specific kind of life-force energy because qi has so many meanings, such as "air," "emotion," and "feelings." Hado literally means "wave motion" or "vibration."

I extend this meaning to define hado as the very air in Mother Nature itself. Hado is everywhere. It is in your house, your office, your plants, your water, even your computer. It fills in empty space as it moves around and is very active. Everything—including you, your pets, the flowers in your garden, and the mug on your desk—is like an antenna that receives hado. After circulating inside the body or other material, hado returns to Mother Nature again.

Hado released from human beings (which I often refer to as "hado energy") contains a tremendous amount of information. It's like a diary and medical chart in one. It tells about emotions, physical status, the past, and even the future. Hado released from inanimate objects tells about the owners, their physical and psychological status, and so on. When hado is consciously released with a purpose, such as healing people, I call it "hado power."

You may be thinking, "Hado is just another way of saying aura, isn't it?" The concepts of hado and aura are somewhat similar. An aura is also released from a person, and you can read information from it. An aura is soft and stays around the body, whereas hado is strong and active, moving constantly. An aura isn't something you intend to release or send, but you can send hado to someone or something with specific purposes once you understand how to use it. Ultimately, hado is able to manipulate the essences of the physical and the intangible. For example, hado can change the taste of food and heal your injuries, and it can also change a person's psyche, such as by turning a severe or aggressive personality into a gentle one.

What Does Hado Look Like?

People perceive hado in various ways. Hado can have an appearance, a density, a temperature, or even a smell. When I see hado, it appears as snow showers with the pale colors of yellow, pink, and blue. When the hado is very powerful, I can see seven rainbow colors, just like the colors in soap bubbles. You may experience it differently.

Hado has its own density, or weight. Some hado is very light and comfortable, and some is very heavy and stifling. Have you ever felt heavy air inside a friend's house? If so, you may have felt the hado released from the house. Many cultures have expressions that use words meaning "heavy" or something similar. I take this to mean that many people actually know the density and heaviness in the air by instinct. Many cultures also have expressions with concepts such as darkness, shadow, and the color black, which they use to express something negative. In Japanese, when we describe people with bad intentions, we say that they have "black stomach." Psychic people of Europe and the Far East see the same black shadow over people. To me, this shows that different cultures have a shared experience and that our sense of hado is universal. Similarly, you may be perceiving the temperature of hado when you use expressions such as "warm-hearted," "warm personality," and so on. I literally sense the temperature rise or fall when I feel certain hado.

The density of the air in a place changes every day, like the weather, because hado circulates; it doesn't stay put. I once taught a client how to perceive the density of hado. After the lesson, he called me from his office. "Something feels wrong with my office today," he said. "I think that one of my secretaries hates me. I sense strange hado around her."

I used my clairvoyant power with hado and told him, "Nobody hates you in the office, Ken. Something personal happened to one of your secretaries last night, and she is a little down today and releasing heavier hado than usual. You didn't feel the difference before, but you have become very sensitive to hado. You will sense things in a different way from now on. Welcome to a new world!"

When my webmaster, Sayuri, was working on my Web site, she tried to scan my photograph and booklet many times, but the scans never came out well; pale yellowish-pink horizontal lines appeared around my head and all over the booklet. Thinking that the scanner was malfunctioning, she decided to give it a break. A few days later, she scanned photographs of other people without any trouble, so she tried my photograph and booklet again. To her surprise, the same yellowish-pink lines appeared. Even the scanner, it seemed, could pick up the hado I am constantly releasing. Also, Sayuri had been working on my book for a while by then; I suppose some of my hado power had been transferred to her, and that led to this incident.

The scanned images were due that day, so Sayuri tried something she had seen me do when I use my hado power with my clients: she put her hand on the scanner and said, "Please cooperate with me and let me scan these clearly because I don't have any more time." Then she tried again. This time, the scans turned out beautifully: the sky behind my head showed a pure blue. Prior to this incident she hadn't been fully convinced about hado, but now she believes there is something in this world that she cannot see.

Hado changes its appearance all the time because of its mobile nature. When people are happy or in a good mood, they release very comfortable and light hado. When I perceive it, it feels just like I am breathing pure oxygen. When people are sad or sick, they release heavy hado. Sometimes I cannot stand the heaviness, so I block it. When people are angry, they send out their hado like steam from a kettle. You probably know what I mean if you've

7

ever seen people who have lost all their strength after they got furious. This is vital energy that is being released, so I try to receive the excess hado and take advantage of it. You feel more energetic when you receive that kind of energy right from the source.

Sources of Hado

Because hado is everywhere, you'll find that just about everything releases it. And the hado is as varied as its source. By nature, everyone has equal access to hado power; however, the output of power is different in each individual, as it goes through our individual bodies. People who are physically and mentally healthy tend to release stronger hado power; in contrast, people who are sick cannot produce much hado power. It's as if their circuits are thinner or even disconnected, resulting in a weaker body. Even if you don't have a lot of hado energy to begin with, you can make it much stronger by training yourself. (I will talk about this in chapter 4.)

Children release very comfortable and pure hado. Previously, I tried to avoid kids in public places as they can be so noisy, but one day I discovered that the hado they release is quite soothing. Now I approach them so that I can benefit from their hado, because pure and comfortable hado has a strong healing power. This may be why elderly people often love to spend time with little children; by experience, they know that they will feel more comfortable when they are with children.

Animals tend to receive rather than release hado, and they are very sensitive to it. When I visit clients, some people are surprised because their pets come close to me and stay next to me. My clients say, "It is strange. My cat never approaches someone she doesn't know. In fact, she usually hides in my bedroom when we have a visitor." Pets feel and enjoy my hado power. They even narrow their eyes, which shows they are totally relaxed. When young and healthy animals release hado, it is usually comfortable hado, similar to children's; it makes sense that elderly or sick people have pet therapy or keep healthy pets in the house.

Dead people release hado, too. Hado from them is released as words, the means of communication with the living. The dead often appear in my session with a client, and they ask me to deliver their message. When my clients get the message right, often both the client and I feel a cold chill or get goosebumps. People in the other world release cold hado when they feel happy. Or my clients may feel something warm come up from deep in their hearts and feel like crying without knowing why. This also means that they get the messages from the departed ones right and cry happy tears for them.

I believe that important religious figures such as Moses, Jesus Christ, Mohammad, and Buddha had very strong hado. Not only did they have the power, but they also fully understood it, which allowed them to perform miracles. Without understanding hado, you cannot reach the truth of the universe, as demonstrated by these religious figures. In ancient times, the air wasn't polluted as it is now, so hado was much stronger because it was purer. Since they received purer hado from Mother Nature, I imagine that those great religious figures could actually do anything: move mountains, walk on water, or heal the sick, as told in many of their stories. Hado power tends to be weakened in polluted air. Naturally, you can benefit more from hado power in places where you enjoy pure air than in larger cities where the air is polluted.

Mother Nature releases different types of energy. Small plants and flowers release weak hado, while large and old trees release very strong hado with healing power. Forests are a great source of hado. The combined energy from big trees works from outside our body to heal us. The ocean also releases one of the greatest amounts of hado, which resonates directly inside our bodies. This is because life comes from the ocean, and the concentration of salt in seawater is the same as that in blood. This may explain why we are drawn to the ocean for rejuvenation. Rivers and lakes release great energy, too, but rivers have stronger hado because their water flow adds mobility, which makes the hado stronger. Hado from the sun is very powerful, as it is from the soil. Soil nourishes plants, trees, flowers, and other life. It's no wonder that people working on farms and nurseries are often healthy and hearty; daily contact with the soil is good for the life force within you.

Every dwelling has its own hado, which is the combined hado from the people who live there; when the people change, the hado changes. Each house has a different hado because the people who reside there imprint their hado into the house all the time. A house with a happy family releases

11

light and comfortable hado; a house with sad people releases heavy hado.

A city releases its own unique hado. By sensing hado from a city and then focusing your own hado, you can actually change it for the better, if only a little. If you live in a city that releases bad hado, you can make improvements by changing the hado around you, such as in your house and in your office. People's perception of hado varies, but I sensed the following when my friend asked me about the hado of several U.S. cities, most of which I have not yet visited. (Please realize that hado changes all the time, like the weather. If you find some of the following comments negative, remember that the city doesn't remain the same all the time.)

I sensed New York City's hado as very strong and active, moving around even at midnight, while cities along the Hudson River on the New Jersey side released rather relaxing hado. Washington, D.C., had very complex hado. I sensed that the bottom layer of the city was kept very neat and clean, but the top part was very dense. The hado from Los Angeles, in contrast, had a very dense layer of hado at the bottom, but it had clean and light hado above the sky. Portland, Oregon, was full of beautiful hado from Mother Nature (such as forests and rivers). Miami released stifling, humid hado. I also sensed people coming out after midnight, smelling of alcohol. San Francisco had heavy hado from cloudy skies, murky water, and sluggish movements. Denver released dark hado. I also saw crime. The snow was tinted and there was a huge gap between the rich and the poor. In Seattle the hado was unclear and stagnant. Compared to other cities, the air was much weaker, as if the city were inside a balloon. (This can be considered a good thing for people who live there, because you can live easily without being affected too much.) Hado was much heavier and solemn in Boston. I saw images of buildings and history; people felt bound by this history and heavy hado. I felt a diversity of people in Dallas, but that the life there was not easy. Compared to other cities, Dallas's hado was much darker. The hado in Atlanta was kind of loose and frivolous. I saw images of workers, but things were left half-finished. Atlanta was almost like another country within the United States.

Each country also releases its own hado. I sensed that the hado from the United States was dynamic and active. I felt the movement of people all over the place, even in the rural areas (most likely because the land is so vast and people have a lot of space to move around in). Japan felt compact and well organized, with limited movement. Germany had hado with history, frugality, firmness, and tall trees. Australia released hado with small houses, simplicity, immigrants, and stiffness. Korea had hado with smells, ego, collectivity, and the strength of wildflowers. England released a hado of high pride, willfulness, and castles. France had hado of alleyways, gray water, and intelligence. China released very interesting hado. The color of hado had become tinted; I think that this was because the country had started to accept the market economy and has been enjoying economic prosperity at the cost of losing some of its culture and traditions. Everything in the world is like a see-saw—a game of balance. If you gain something, you lose something.

Technically, outer space does not have air, but I sense that a totally different type of hado from another dimension has filled the empty space. I believe that it is extremely pure, which makes it extremely powerful. I have heard stories about astronauts who became philosophers or more spiritual after returning from space. I am not surprised. Because they were exposed to that powerful hado, their lives have changed and they are open to other dimensions.

How Hado Interacts

Because hado is a wave vibration, when one hado meets another, there are three ways in which they can influence each other: rebounding, resonation, and absorption.

When hado is released, it rebounds. Imagine that you have to work with a person you don't like very much. Your hado will rebound no matter how hard you pretend to like her; naturally, she senses that you don't like her, and her hado rebounds, too. This happens to me on occasion; sometimes I must counsel people whom I don't care for, but I have to send my hado power to them because it is my job. In such cases, I try to send my hado power from a distance.

When you meet someone you love and who loves you back, your hado and the hado from your loved one resonate. They integrate and become stronger. Picture it like snowflake particles, very active and reflecting their mutual happiness. I believe this is why a happy couple becomes similar after a long marriage: the individual hado mix and integrate all the time, and each influences the other's energy.

The output of hado is different in every individual. When a person with strong hado meets a person with weak hado, the weaker hado absorbs the stronger. When I meet old or sick people, they absorb my hado like dry sponges. However, one hado never negates another; there is always feedback from the weaker to the stronger, no matter how weak it is.

Hado can also be blocked. I sometimes encounter clients whose minds are closed to hado, and they purposely block mine out. Blocking is also a technique you can use to protect yourself from bad hado. When you must go to a place or meet people who release bad hado, block yourself so that they cannot influence you. You don't need any special technique; just be determined to not be affected by it. Try thinking, "Bad hado cannot come close to me!" or, as I like to say, "Resolute!" Some people can block themselves effectively if they imagine beautiful light from above embracing and protecting them; others visualize a firm shell covering and shielding their body.

Hado can be so powerful that it moves objects. One day when I was at home with friends, I received a call from a woman seeking advice about a relationship. After talking with her for a brief time, I realized that she was only hoping to improve the situation in an egotistic manner, and her attitude made me angry. First I tried to reason with her, but she wouldn't listen to me at all. Finally I lost control, raised my voice, and said, "Don't you think that you are being much too selfish?" Simultaneously, a pair of earrings that I had put on the table near the phone flew off and hit the wall. One of my friends picked them up and gasped, "Look, your earrings are totally bent. Your anger made the earrings blow off!" After this happened, I tried hard to control my feelings and vowed that I would never let this kind of thing happen again. (Of course, my friends still tease me about the incident.)

Mechanisms of Hado

Our world is filled with hado that moves around all the time. Hado enters all things on the earth, circulates inside the material, and then returns to the air. When hado goes through materials, both the hado and the material are changed; in other words, hado leaves its own essences in the material, and the material adds its own characteristics to the hado while it circulates inside. After hado returns to the air in Mother Nature, the influence of the material is diluted and purified.

As long as it circulates, hado remains light and pure. However, when hado becomes stagnant, it gets heavier and more negative; therefore, it is very important to make an exit for hado in closed spaces such as houses, apartments, and offices in order to move and exchange the air inside. Just as you wouldn't use the same water for washing and rinsing when doing laundry, you don't want the same hado circulating continuously. You can create exits in houses and closed spaces by opening doors, windows, and ventilators. Window screens block hado, so be sure to open the screens when you want to exchange the air. Turn on a fan and let old air exit the space and fresh air enter. You can also use a feather duster to move the air.

People ask me where hado comes from. In people, hado comes from the heart. When you think of or care for someone or something, hado is released and sent directly to the person or thing you are thinking of. So hado can easily be sent directly to a person or an object or from a remote place. When

I am asked to send hado remotely, I concentrate to feel hado from that person or thing. I don't even have to know their names or where they are; for some reason, I can be connected with them accurately, without any mistakes. Then I start to feel them right in front of me, as if there were a worm hole that directly connected me to them, and I start to send my hado power to them. Therefore, there is no difference if the person is in front of me or far away. In this respect, hado is very much like prayer. The following story will illustrate what I mean.

I was visiting a hospital, and I noticed an old man with lung disease who was coughing all the time. Although he was a stranger to me, it was painful to see him coughing, so I prayed for his recovery whenever I could. After a while, I realized that he was not coughing anymore. I asked a nurse what had happened to him, and she told me that his condition had improved dramatically and he was going to be discharged. I had sent my hado energy to this old man simply by hoping for his recovery. Your prayers reach the people you are praying for in the form of hado, which protects them from danger and minimizes their suffering.

Hado can also be likened to electricity. When hado works for someone or something, it is like a switch turns on inside the body. The strength of each person's or object's hado is as variable as electricity; some hado has the strength of static, some of thunder. In fact, hado and electricity are closely connected. When I use hado power or when dead people are sending hado energy to communicate with us, electric appliances often react and start to flicker.

One day I visited a house filled with dark and heavy hado, and I started to move the air in the living room by sending my hado power. Everybody in the room scattered because the huge chandelier began to flicker and move; that's where the heavy hado was stagnating and where I sent my hado power.

Another time, the lights in my bedroom started to make a buzzing sound. When I left my bedroom, I could hear that the noise had stopped. I entered the room again, and the noise started again. The lights must be reacting to some part of my body, I thought, but I didn't know where in my body it could be. Six months later, I visited a doctor and found out I had a gallstone. I immediately knew that the gallstone was the source of the buzzing sound I had been hearing. As I had expected, the noise stopped after the gallstone was removed.

Some people ask me if hado can be switched on and off, like electricity. When I send my hado power into something, I need to be focused on it; you could say I "switch on" my hado power. When I feel heavy hado energy around me and it is too much to bear, I can switch off my ability so that I don't have to be influenced by negative energy; however, my normal state is to be releasing hado energy, even when I am sleeping. When I stay in a hotel, the air in my room becomes light just because I am sleeping there overnight. Objects are also affected by the hado I continuously release. I received an old ring from a friend and put it away because it was a bit too worn out for my taste. A year or so later, when I remembered the ring, I took it out and found that it had become as shiny as a brand-new ring. I wore it to see what my friend would say. She didn't recognize the ring at all; she just said, "What a beautiful ring! Where did you get it?"

Hado and electricity are linked in my mind for another reason. Only a few centuries ago, nobody knew about electricity. If you were to travel back in time and tell people from the eighteenth century that an unseen energy called "electricity" would give light, they would think you were out of your mind. Hado in the early twenty-first century is the same as electricity in the eighteenth. Not many people can see or sense it yet, but some-day—hopefully, very soon—it will be understood by many people.

II

Applications
of Hado

波動

The concept of hado is very simple, similar to the truth of the universe. The truth is always simple. Einstein reached a simple formula, $E = mc^2$, after years of long calculation. Please do not make hado complicated as you try to grasp it, because you have always known it by instinct; it is the natural course of things. Try to understand it with a child's pure heart. If you can feel it and accept it, you can make miracles happen, too.

Now that you have some background in the basic concept of hado, I will explain the many applications of hado and how I use this power to help my clients.

Hado and Inanimate Objects

The source of hado is our heart—our thoughts and emotions—and strong hado flows down to weaker hado; therefore, inanimate objects tend to receive people's hado. When enough hado is imprinted on an inanimate object, it starts to have its own energy, or heart. The longer and closer the object stays with people, the more hado will be imprinted on it and the stronger that hado will become.

I drive a car every day to visit my clients. Since my car receives my strong hado energy all the time, my friends tell me that they can feel a kind of personality from it and from a car I once owned. When I had to drive a long distance, I would picture a look of exhaustion on it, just like in a cartoon. When I asked it to run a little more, I would see it clenching its teeth to go farther. When I arrived home, I would see its face relax, and it would start to go to sleep in no time. I felt sorry for my car in those situations. One day it seemed to me that my car's face had become really old, and I sensed that long drives were too painful for it. I sold the car to someone who would keep the car in good condition and who wouldn't take it on long drives.

After using or keeping something for a while, it may start to have a "consciousness" or "awareness" from receiving your hado energy; therefore, it is important to treat everything with care. One of my clients told me that someone in her office has a "magic touch" with computers. When a computer crashes or is infected with a virus, everybody runs to him for help. Of course, the person has a deep knowledge of computers; but according to her, that is not the only reason people ask him for help. When he does something simple, such as restarting the computer, it works normally again. If she does the same thing, the computer still has problems. This person likely has hado power that is especially good for computers or machines. The next time your computer breaks and you can't find someone with the magic touch, try asking the computer to cooperate with you. The machine may have a slight consciousness, and it just may work for you.

Some objects are more susceptible to hado and tend to absorb stronger hado. Jewelry in particular has this absorbing tendency. You might feel that your jewelry has lost its original sparkle after you've worn it for a while. What's happened is that your jewelry has absorbed your negative energy. My clients are usually extremely exhausted and have serious problems when they come to see me. I often find that their jewelry has absorbed their negative energy and is exhausted, too. In some cases, the jewelry has started to release negative energy back to the owner, because it has reached its capacity. In such cases, I ask my clients to put their jewelry on the table, and I send my hado power into it and let the negative energy out. Usually my clients get very excited because their jewelry starts to sparkle right in front of their eyes.

Some of them even forget about their original problems and bring in more jewelry for cleaning at the next session!

A client came to see me to for a health problem and left feeling much lighter and with a much better complexion after receiving my hado. At the next session, she brought her wedding ring, which was terribly bent. She told me that she had had a slight pain on her finger during our first session; then on the way back home, the pain had become unbearable, and she had looked at her finger. To her surprise, the ring she wore was bending, and she took off the ring in a hurry. In front of her eyes, the ring twisted completely, as if it had been waiting for her to take it off. It seemed the ring had been absorbing Julia's bad hado because of her sickness, and it bent because it could handle no more.

A friend bought a beautiful ring from an antique shop. I noticed that the density of the air around the ring was very heavy, so I asked her, "Don't you feel something has changed since you bought the ring? I feel like the ring is avoiding contact with men." She looked at me in surprise and said that men hadn't spent time with her ever since she bought the ring. I used my clairvoyant power with hado to see through the ring's past. It appeared to me as a woman's engagement ring; however, the former owner's fiancé had left her and married another woman. The owner of the ring became very desperate and felt that she would never trust men again. Her hatred toward men was released from her in the form of negative hado and imprinted very deeply into the ring. Many decades had passed since then, but the ring remained full of hatred. When this negative hado becomes too strong, people refer to an object as being "cursed." The men around my friend must have sensed that strong negative hado and felt uncomfortable around her. I advised her to sell the ring; she reported to me later that her life had gone back to normal after she had given it away.

You may be familiar with the famous Hope Diamond, the huge blue jewel exhibited at the National Museum of Natural History in Washington, D.C. It might be the most notorious diamond in history; many people who owned it experienced tragic deaths, including Louis XVI and Marie Antoinette, who were both executed during the French Revolution. Although I have never seen it, I can't help but think that it is cursed; it has been absorbing human emotions, including very negative ones, for centuries.

Positive hado can be imprinted on inanimate objects just as easily as negative hado. You may find that a gift from someone who has passed away comes into your life unexpectedly. If you receive such a gift, please keep it because the gift will protect you; those gifts are filled with love from the departed one, even if you didn't have a chance to interact with him or her while he or she were alive. I once communicated with a departed person during a session I had with his granddaughter-in-law. He said that he would give a gift—something sweet—to this woman because she had taken such good care of her father-in-law and he was grateful for it. I told my client that soon she would receive something sweet unexpectedly. Later the client told me that she received a special Japanese snack from remote relatives she hadn't heard from in years.

We have special bonds with others and are linked by fate. Dead people may ask you to remember them sometimes or to be friends with their family. Please thank them and pray for their peace in the other world, tell them that you understand their message, and promise them that you will treat the gift with care. Remembrance will be your strongest charm.

From my experience, objects that have a long history, such as masterpieces, have more than a heart; they have a spirit. When you have a chance to deal with an object like this, you must take extra care since it has a strong personality and sometimes even a high sense of pride. An orchestral musician once showed me her prized possession: a violin. I had heard that it was a famous masterpiece; however, something about it bothered me. I said, "I understand that this violin has belonged to many master musicians. I sense that it picked up many habits from them. Do you feel this violin almost turns away from you?"

"How did you know? I feel exactly that way. I cannot create a good sound with it. Actually, I think I am in trouble." She looked as though she didn't know what to do with this masterpiece.

I picked up the hado released from the violin just by observing the way she handled it. The violin was indeed a masterpiece. It had its own heart and spirit, with a strong personality and attitude. It had belonged to many great musicians, but none of them had been able to make full use of it. The violin felt that Jane didn't reach its level of performance. That's why it turned away from her.

I told her truthfully what I felt, and I advised her, "Before a performance, in a humble way, ask the violin to cooperate with you, even though you aren't experienced enough to play it. And if it is possible, try to sell it to someone who can make full use of it." She followed my advice, and she told me that she could make much better sound from it by asking the violin for its cooperation.

Inanimate objects often will suddenly break or disappear, as if sacrificing themselves for us. Before I visited New York for the first time, I had a feeling that something bad would happen to me, such as getting the flu or having trouble with the hotel. Right before the trip, the windshield of my car cracked while I was driving on the highway. The repair cost a lot of money, but I knew that the glass had cracked itself for me so that I could avoid major trouble during the trip.

A client of mine was once at an airport when a bottle broke and spilled wine on her clothing. She was totally embarrassed because she had to travel in stained clothes; however, in view of this theory, she probably avoided other trouble at her destination. During another trip, I saw a friend lose fifty dollars in a strange way. While we were riding in a taxi, she put the money into her pocket, and five minutes later, the money was gone. Of course, before we left the taxi, we searched everywhere in the backseat but we couldn't find the money. I told her that the money had disappeared from her pocket so that she could avoid problems at our destination. It's my belief that there is a link between these occurrences and our unconscious mind, and that's why things break down or disappear for us.

A similar phenomenon you may have experienced is that computers or electric appliances will malfunction or break down when their owner develops some physical infirmity. These technologies are sensitive to the hado released from the person who touches them, and they absorb his or her illness through the electrical circuits. When they reach their capacity, they break down. A friend told me that two new computers in her office had broken down in only three months, and her boss was not happy about it. Even the technicians couldn't figure out why it was happening. Her boss said that if a third one broke down, they would suspect that Nina had done something to break the computers; however, there was no third time. She developed irritable bowel syndrome and had to take sick leave. She remembered my stories of things breaking down on behalf of people and thanked the two computers that broke down for her.

The next time something suddenly breaks or disappears, take time to consider why it has happened. Did you avoid a negative experience, or did it alert you to a medical problem? If you think something has broken on your behalf, you might want to thank it. Or if your electric appliances break down often, it might be a good idea to schedule regular checkups for yourself.

When something important disappears or breaks or when something unusual happens, it could also be a sign. A sign tells you about an important turning point or transition in your life. You often don't realize it until after the fact, but you can tell it's a sign if a significant event happens and then something bigger happens. In my case, I lost very special rings twice in my life: one was a sign of divorce; the other was a sign of my son's death. Also, the colors of a Japanese folding screen in my living room suddenly started to fade; that was also a sign of my son's death. Of course, there are many positive signs, too. Look back on any signs that may have occurred before a major event in your life. This will help you clue in to the signs appearing before you today. As you begin to recognize signs more easily, you will be more prepared for what follows a sign and can experience it fully.

How *Hado* Manipulates the Essence of a Material

Hado circulates everywhere on the earth. All things on the earth are part of this circulation, receiving and releasing hado continuously as if they are breathing. When hado enters into something, it can manipulate the essence of that material.

Some clients are skeptical of my hado power. When this happens, I ask clients to fill two glasses with tap water and taste them both. Of course, they taste the same. Then I send my hado power to only one glass and then ask my clients to taste the water from both glasses again. They react with surprise because one of the glasses tastes the same as before, but the one that received my hado power tastes like expensive mineral water. If my clients are still not totally convinced, I ask them to keep both glasses and see what happens. Later they report that the one that received my hado power stays as it is much longer than the one without hado, which goes bad.

When I visited Oregon, I made a different presentation using wine. This time, I did the experiment the other way around. First, I sent my hado power into the wine and asked everyone to taste it. They all said that the wine tasted more like grape juice than wine. (For some reason, alcohol always disappears when hado touches liquor.) Then I brought the original taste back into the wine and asked them to taste again. Everyone almost spit it out, because the alcohol and the original sweetness were returned to the wine, and it was a very bad and cheap wine!

I did another experiment remotely. From my house, I sent my hado power to one particular beer bottle in a friend's refrigerator. In my mind, I pointed to one beer bottle carefully and focused on it so that the other bottles would not be affected. After sending adequate hado power, I phoned him.

"I just sent my hado power to a beer bottle at the right front corner on the second shelf. The other bottles did not receive my hado power. Taste the difference and call me back."

First my friend wondered how I knew where the beer bottles were located, but he said he would do it. He called me back after a while and told me that he was with his friends, and all of them were astonished because the taste of the beer that had received my hado tasted totally different—like an expensive beer.

You've likely experienced this on some level. Have you ever thought that you were following a famous chef's recipe exactly, but the taste was not the same? Even if you are cooking something very simple, such as eggs, using the exact same ingredients, have you found that someone else's eggs are much more delicious and wondered why? The answer is simple: All good chefs have strong hado. They release it without realizing it and manipulate the taste of food by touching it. The next time you cook, think about me so that you will be connected to me and receive my hado power. You will be surprised when your ordinary food is transformed into something very special.

People sometimes ask me if eating meat is bad for you or it it has a negative effect on hado. I have never felt that way. I eat meat often because using hado power requires a lot of energy, and for me, meat is a very good source of those energies.

Everything in the life cycle has its own fate. I think animals accept their fates because they have pure hearts, although the law of Mother Nature can be very cruel to them. The most important thing for us is to be thankful to animals or plants for offering their lives for us and not to waste them. If you eat meat with appreciation, the spirits of the animals will rest in peace.

Hado and Place

Good hado feels light and comfortable, circulating all the time. As the source of hado is people's hearts, good hado is filled with love and good will. Bad hado feels heavy, stifling, and stagnant. Bad hado is full of negative emotions, such as hatred, sorrow, pain, and jealousy.

A place may have some spots with good hado and some with bad. For example, in a shopping mall, some shops may have many customers and others may not. If you take a good look at each shop, you will find that shops with many customers always have good hado. Good hado naturally attracts people because it feels comfortable; bad hado pushes people away because it makes them feel uneasy.

Mother Nature is filled with good hado purified by big trees, oceans, forests, the sun, and soil. Graves, museums with ancient relics, human skeletons, ruins, and old castles release bad hado because they are full of thoughts and emotions of people who have passed away, which makes the air heavy. On the other hand, ashes of loved ones kept in your home never release bad hado. Non-family members' remains may release bad hado because the dead feel that you're invading their peace, as if you were entering their home without knocking. When people die, their spirit passes on to another world, but their last thoughts and emotions linger in our world. They are usually imprinted on things that the dead were attached to or to the place where they died. If a person's last thought was a painful one, it becomes heavy hado and lingers. If you cannot avoid visiting places with heavy hado, block yourself by thinking, "Bad hado cannot come close to me" so you don't have to be influenced by the heavy energy.

Places of worship release special hado. When people worship something, it actually becomes a deity, as the hado from worshippers goes into the person or thing and imprints their thoughts and emotions on it. The more people worship it, the more hado is absorbed, and it starts to have its own heart. Also, as people spend time praying, their prayers transform into a collective divine hado. After absorbing divine hado for a long time, a place becomes the home of gods; therefore, it's important to be respectful of places of worship and to never visit religious sites simply for amusement.

You can change bad hado into good hado. Since bad hado has lost its mobility, you can help it circulate with a fan that blows toward windows or doors. When bad hado reaches Mother Nature again, it is diluted and purified. I was once admitted to a hospital, and I spent half a day cleansing the hado inside my room because it was filled with all the negative hado left by previous patients. After the operation, when the nurses asked me to move to another room, I felt like crying because I knew that I would have to cleanse the hado there! It is especially important to cleanse the hado in an environment like a hospital, where patients have died, so that bad hado does not linger and affect other people.

If you or a loved one has to stay in the hospital, you can avoid the effects of negative hado by opening windows (if possible) and doors and trying to move the air in the room. Also, when you clean the hado in the room, try to visualize me so that you can be connected to me. If you are visiting a patient, try to drop by a park or have some contact with nature prior to entering the hospital room. Bringing the strong hado of nature to the hospital is sure to help. And the most important thing to do is to pray for the recovery of the patient whenever you can. Your prayer surely reaches your loved ones, and it makes a big difference in recovery.

A few years ago, I used these techniques in a number of restaurants in Japan whose owners were worried that their customers' fear of mad cow disease would hurt their business. People working in the beef industry suffered when cases of the disease were reported in Japan, and a lot of steak and barbeque restaurants were forced to close. At that time, some restaurants asked me to send my hado power into their businesses. As a result, all the restaurants I was involved with survived.

Hado can tell you the character or potential of houses, apartments, or other dwellings. A couple once asked me to examine the house they were planning to buy because they had reservations about it. I went to the house accompanied by the couple and the real estate agent. It was a rather small house but the facade looked solid. When we reached the kitchen, I shouted in surprise. I had seen a burst of flame. My body stiffened, and I asked everybody to stay quiet. I started to send hado power to the flame.

Then I had a vision of an unknown married couple that argued in the kitchen every day. I told the agent, "I think the previous owners had a bad relationship and had terrible quarrels. That's one of the reasons they had to sell their house. They released so much strong negative energy with their anger."

Despite this, the couple really liked the house. "OK, I understand," I said. "You won't have any problem if I send hado power to the house from now on." Soon the fire became smaller and smaller and finally disappeared. The anger was removed from the kitchen. The couple bought the house and still live there happily to this day.

I have experienced many similar cases. For example, after moving into a new place, a couple starts to quarrel badly, children have trouble concentrating on their work, or the husband hardly ever comes home. In those cases, hado released from previous owners may be imprinted in the rooms and may be affecting the new occupants' lives.

Land is alive, too. When I visited a piece of land with a leveled surface, I suddenly had a vision of a big fire. I asked my client who took me there if there had been a fire at the location. He said, "How did you know this? That's why I asked you to come here. I want to buy this land but I feel uneasy about it. I heard that whenever people build a house or building here, there's a fire and they end up selling. What do you think?"

I focused on the location further; there had been a big fire about a century ago, and I thought that some people had lost their lives. The land had remembered all this and had suffered from the experience. I sent my hado power carefully, and I told the land that the fire happened more than a century ago, so it didn't have to suffer any longer. Later, my client bought that land and still lives there peacefully without any problems.

When you are looking for an apartment or a house, it is very important to choose one with good hado because it directly affects your life. Please bring this book and visualize me when you are looking for a new place to live and get a feeling for the place without any judgment. If it doesn't feel right or my face in the photograph looks sad, I recommend that you not take that property.

Hado and Clairvoyance

Hado opens the door to clairvoyant abilities. Since I have had this ability my entire life, it is difficult for me to describe how I tap into this power. It is like asking a composer how she writes music. Hado is something I actually feel in the air. You can become clairvoyant as you practice hado, but you may not perceive it as I do; everyone's experience is unique. If you would like to explore your clairvoyant power, all I can advise is that you learn to quiet your mind, become sensitive to your hunches, and be open to where this exploration takes you.

I'd like to share some stories from my experience of using hado to see clairvoyantly.

A businessman named Mr. Tanaka once visited me for a consultation. "I'd like to know what you see in these," he said as he held out some business cards. "They are all important business partners."

I put the business cards on the table and used my clairvoyant power to visualize them one by one. First I looked at a business card, and then I started to sense that a certain part was heavier than the others. I concentrated further and started to see a human figure in the card. In this case, I felt that the middle of the body was heavier than the rest and saw a dark shadow on it. I asked myself if it was revealing a problem with the person's internal organs or the person's heart. It turned out to be the latter.

"I see that this person is black-hearted. I wonder what this blackness means. Will he try to cheat you or . . ."

Unfortunately, Mr. Tanaka had already been cheated. This person had already been deported from Japan for his offense, but Mr. Tanaka kept his business card, hoping to collect the debt, as it was a large sum of money.

The next business card troubled me. "I see blackness over his legs. Tell this person to be careful." Three months later this person was in a car accident that injured his legs.

I picked up another business card. It was one of his employees, and I saw his legs moving around. "What is this person's job? Is he in sales?"

Mr. Tanaka said, "He is our administrative officer. The reason why I brought this card is that he hasn't looked happy lately, and I feel that he's going to quit."

I advised him, "Why don't you give him a chance to do sales? He is very active and he cannot stand to stay in an office all day. He loves to be on the road and traveling."

With the fourth business card, I saw blackness over a man's mouth, but the air was circulating. I found it interesting, so I focused on feeling the hado from his mouth. The air felt comfortable and light, which means that his mouth brings money in business affairs. But I also felt uneasy.

I advised him, "He has a big mouth. Not many people trust him, but he'll bring you a big business opportunity in the near future. If you could manage him, he'd bring you big money." Mr. Tanaka looked doubtful but somehow he knew what I was trying to tell him. I sensed his hado with joy.

Mr. Suzuki, an unemployed man in his forties, came to me for advice because he was planning to set up a new gravestone store, using his former experience as a gravestone salesman for a large corporation.

"Will this shop be successful?" he asked me.

Suddenly, a particular Buddhist temple came to my mind. The temple is located by the side of the road I usually drive on, and for some reason, it seemed to me to be shining brightly all the time. I wrote down the name and directions to the temple and gave them to him. "I don't know anyone at this temple, but go seek counsel with the priest about your new business. I visualize the priest and you cleaning the temple together with delight."

He visited the temple immediately and he spoke to the priest about his business plan. The priest was willing to offer him his advice.

While preparing for the opening of the gravestone store, Mr. Suzuki continued to visit the priest. One day the priest said to him, "There's another temple with which I am associated. From what I can tell, you would be a great priest. I recommend that you perform the ascetic training to become a Buddhist monk. If you do, I'll take care of all the expenses until you accomplish this."

The words of the priest touched the man's heart so deeply that he gratefully accepted this unexpected and generous offer. The ascetic training is going well, and Mr. Suzuki is satisfied with his fulfilling new life.

As you can see, hado can give you information about the past, present, and future. It also can tell you about people's compatibility.

I was invited to a wedding reception, and for some reason, I felt reluctant to go. I attended the party anyway. At the reception, I was unexpectedly asked to sing for the guests. As a professional vocalist, I couldn't decline, so I asked a pianist to accompany me. Strangely enough, I couldn't hear the piano at all. As you can imagine, my song was a disaster. The newlyweds and their relatives and friends all looked at me in a miserable way, not knowing what to say. I wondered why I couldn't hear the piano. Later, I thought the hado energy at the reception might have interfered with the sound of the piano so that it couldn't reach my ears. I took this as a bad sign. Not long after, I heard that the newlywed couple divorced right after the honeymoon.

One day a flutist visited me and told me about a nightmare she had had. "In my dream, I played and played but no sound came out of my flute. That made me very nervous. Please send hado energy into me so that I can play the flute without any worries at my upcoming concert."

While I sent the hado into her, I used clairvoyant power and received a vision. "I see a gentle flow of a river. Don't worry. The concert will be successful."

48

She gasped. "How can you know about that? One of the tunes I play has a motif of 'a gentle flow of a river.' I am so surprised!"

I guaranteed that the concert would be a success and told her to enjoy playing the flute with confidence, but she was not yet convinced. "Would you come and send hado energy into me before the concert?"

As promised, I visited her rehearsal hall and sent hado energy into her and her instrument. While I observed their rehearsal, her students said things like, "Sounds much better!" and "I think the sound has improved." I had the same impression of her playing. Of course, the sound wouldn't be improved only by sending hado to her, but I assume that my client prepared herself for playing the flute by receiving my hado, and it improved her concentration level as well. Furthermore, her self-confidence played a large part in her success: she believed everything would be just fine because she received the hado energy.

A woman with a look of exhaustion came to see me for advice. "I have a daughter living in Los Angeles," she said. "She has suffered so much because her husband is beating her, and she fears that one day she will be killed. If I were in Los Angeles, I could help her somehow, but I cannot do anything from here. Please help my daughter."

I sent my hado power into her daughter and received information clairvoyantly. "Your son-in-law is hitting your daughter because he has a fear of losing her," I said. "If she tries to escape now, things could get worse. From now on, I will continue to send hado power into your daughter to protect her from the violence, and into your son-in-law to be able to contain his anger. But please give me a little more time and be patient. Also keep me posted on the developments in their relationship."

I continued sending hado power to the woman in Los Angeles, and then a month later, the mother called me and said, "Thank you so much for your help. My daughter says her husband's violence has almost stopped."

I was relieved to hear this, but I told her, "It's time for your daughter to file for divorce. I will continue to send hado power so that she can get divorced safely. Again, please inform me of how it goes."

Two more months passed. Then I heard good news from the mother that the daughter's divorce was approved and that she had returned home safely.

Hado power can also be used to discover a child's hidden talent.

One day a mother and daughter visited me. "My daughter is suffering from terrible dermatitis," the girl's mother said. "Is there any way you can treat her?" The somber sixteen-year-old girl's neck was inflamed.

Using hado power, something suddenly came to my mind. I could feel it in the air that the girl's skin problem could be healed by singing lessons. I asked the daughter, "Do you like singing?"

Her face brightened, and she answered, "Yes, I love it!"

I told the mother to treat her daughter's dermatitis with vocal lessons, not by medicine or sending hado power. She looked doubtful. "Is that true? Does she really have that kind of talent?"

"It is understandable that parents can miss their children's hidden talents. By listening to her voice, I can clearly hear her gift of song."

After considering my suggestion, the mother asked that I give her daughter vocal lessons. Soon the girl showed her exceptional talent, and her dermatitis was healed in no time. The girl's stress and blocked energy had flared up in the form of a skin affliction. Singing released the stagnant hado, and the active, strong, positive hado began circulating freely. As she decreased her stress and built strong self-confidence, she started to get better grades at school, and passed the college entrance examination for the singing course in a breeze.

Children are full of hado energy, and they have to release it in a relaxed way, a way they can truly enjoy. If parents are too strict about a child's discipline, the child cannot release energy well, which can lead to physical symptoms. Everybody has his or her own fate, and I see it in people's faces, especially children's because children are so pure and have no intention of hiding or faking things, and their hado flows so smoothly. I feel powerless when I see a painful fate in a newborn's face. If parents do what they can to find and nurture the real talent hidden inside, such children can have a dream and a hope that will give them strength to cope with their fate. A supportive environment that encourages children and their special hado is important for every family.

Hado and Healing

Just as hado power can manipulate the essences of materials, it can do the same for the human mind and body. People call this healing. Most of my current clients visit me for this purpose.

I often tell a client to visit a doctor before seeing me. I do this when I sense that the symptom is hidden and not yet fully revealed. People often don't take simple steps to heal themselves, such as getting enough rest and eating well, until they know for sure that they are sick and see undeniable signs (especially if they lead busy or stressful lives). Hado power tends to reveal symptoms and problems that are hidden inside, and I don't want to upset my clients by naming symptoms. Another reason I advise a visit to a doctor is that I want to see the client's condition through the doctor's eyes. In other words, a third party's diagnosis helps me—and my client—chart the progress through the healing process. We can see the hado working by markers, such as cholesterol level, tumor size, and so on. Also, I have found that people with diseases such as cancer, especially in the advanced stages, are healed much faster when the tumor is surgically removed and hado power is used to focus on the recovery process. Hado is most effective during recovery and during the early stages of cancer. It can be helpful before surgery, as it can gather the cells that are spread out over a large area and make it easier for surgeons to cut the tumor out. We should all use common sense when using hado. It is not magic and should not be used to replace conventional medicine; however, the results can be miraculous when the conditions are right.

As I have described, when something is wrong with a person, I usually sense that the air around the affected area is heavy and dense, just like a black shadow. For example, when I see somebody with a liver problem, I usually have a vision of the shape of a liver with heaviness. The heavier the part is, the more severe the illness is. At other times, I see a light and pure hado that brings good luck.

Healing with hado can be accomplished either in person or remotely. This is another good thing about hado: people who benefit from it don't even have to know that someone is sending the power to them. Remote healing can work just as well as hands-on healing. The only difference between direct and remote hado power is that direct hado is softer and wider, mostly sent by touching through hands and fingers; in contrast, remote hado is sharper, has more speed, and goes directly into the spot that needs healing.

I used to feel more confident doing direct healing because I receive instant feedback from the recipient. Sending hado directly to a patient in front of me, I receive hado energy back from the patient. When I began practicing remote healing, I would ask my clients to keep me posted because I was less sure of its effectiveness. Now, however, I am fully confident in this power, and I don't need any more updates. Actually, I prefer remote to direct healing because direct healing takes a toll on me, physically. Feedback from the sick can be very heavy, and my energy is depleted for a few days after being exposed to it. I don't receive this feedback when I use remote healing; also, I'm able to use my time more effectively, sending hado power to more people who need it.

Hado works even when sent unintentionally. One day a friend called me about her father's illness; strangely enough, the sickness disappeared as soon as I received her call. It seems that when the information about her father came to me, he was immediately connected and received my hado power instantly.

Some people are very sensitive to hado healing and can be healed after only a few sessions. Others need at least six months to see an improvement in their condition. One of the readers of my first booklet fell into the former category. "I thought that your hado booklet would bring me something very special," she said. "However, the day I read the booklet, I had a terrible food poisoning incident and couldn't stop vomiting for three days."

"Do you feel that your body became cleaner and lighter?" I asked her. "I can tell that your body is very sensitive to hado power."

At that point, she hadn't noticed a change, but later she told me that her drinking behavior dramatically changed after the food poisoning. In the past, she often did not know when to stop drinking and ended up with terrible hangovers. But after the food poisoning, she no longer wanted to have more than two drinks. Her relationship with alcohol was changed forever. It seems that the negative thoughts and feelings that dwelled deep inside her for years were released by the hado power, and this hidden illness came to light after receiving it. I believe that if she had kept her stress inside of her stomach, she would have had stomach cancer or a stomach-related illness in the future.

I see similarities when I work on people with alcohol or drug problems and those with mental illness. There is something hidden inside that has to be revealed and brought to the surface; otherwise, the client cannot be healed. I always tell the client's family that the symptoms will get worse before they get better. This can be shocking for both the client and the client's family, and the client needs the family's full support during the treatment.

One August night, a vocal student visited me about her sick mother. She knew I was an advisor at a senior care facility, but she didn't know anything about my hado power. Her mother was too weak to swallow and could only have fluid food. The doctors told my student that her mother wouldn't survive past October unless something was done. They scheduled an operation for mid-September to make an incision in her stomach and insert a tube to administer nutrients directly.

I told her about hado power for the first time and promised to send it to her mother immediately. As she didn't know anything about hado, she looked puzzled and not at all convinced by what I said; however, after the student left my house, I sent my hado power to her mother anyway.

The next morning, I received a call from my student. She said, "Ms. Matsuzaki, something very unusual happened this morning. My mother was able to swallow normal food! I wasn't convinced about your hado power last night, but I thank you so much for whatever you have done for my mother. I never expected that my mother would eat again." Shortly after this, the operation was cancelled.

Another client came to see me about her pre-cancer status. I asked her to sit down and started to send my hado power by touching her. I had a vision of a small tumor in her breast, but I strongly felt that it would disappear because it was so small and hadn't turned into cancer yet. Fortunately, I found her body very susceptible to hado power. I was assured that she would be OK.

After sending enough hado power to her, I gave her my photograph and said, "Whenever you have time, please touch the area where you have the tumor and visualize me by using this picture. You can be connected to me and you will receive my hado power." She promised me that she would practice this every day.

I heard great news from her in a month. She had had a lumpectomy but the result showed no trace of the tumor. Strangely enough, her doctor could not even find any scar tissue from the previous needle biopsy. Hado power had worked at the cellular level and healed her.

I have experienced many similar cases: One of my clients had an ovarian tumor that disappeared within a couple of days after I sent my hado power. Another client's prolonged lung cancer disappeared within a day after I sent my hado power. In both cases, doctors double- and triple-checked their X-rays and told their patients that they had no idea why this had happened. Both clients told me that they had had terrible pain while they were receiving my hado power. Hado is not magic; therefore patients sometimes suffer from the pain of dynamic recovery. I imagine that their cells were rapidly moving around with my hado power to demolish the cancer cells, and this caused the severe pain. The difference between people who are susceptible to the healing power of hado and those who are not is in their cells. Genetics, of course, is an important factor for the plasticity of cells. The cells of those who are sensitive to hado are somewhat softer. Hard cells are less attuned to hado; they are not on the same wavelength, and it takes longer to feel the effects of hado. This plasticity makes all the difference in receptiveness and the speed of recovery.

Self-Healing

Some people wonder if I experience physical problems; the answer is yes, of course. At such times, I visit doctors and take the medications they prescribe, and I also use my hado power to heal myself. For example, if I am having trouble with my stomach, I visualize my stomach in front of me and send hado into the affected area. Or if I need to see a dentist, I will send hado power into the dentist before treatment so that he or she won't make any mistakes, and then I send hado power into myself. When I am sick and feeling exhausted, I simply don't have the power to heal myself, because using hado takes a lot of energy. At those times, I try to get lots of rest.

Children and Healing

Usually, children can be healed in a short period of time—in some cases, almost instantly. I attribute this to the fact that they are innocent and have pure hearts, never block their minds or hearts to hado, and have young, soft cells that let hado power work quickly. When I send my hado power directly into children, they laugh. Once I asked a child why she was giggling, and she said she felt something moving around her body and it tickled.

When I'm visited by a mother whose child suffers from a chronic illness, I teach the mother how to use hado power, because nothing is stronger than a mother's love.

One night a mother whose child had serious pneumonia called me and asked for my help. The child had a high fever, and the doctor said that he was not sure the child would make it through the night; even if he did make it, he might suffer permanent consequences. I sent my hado power to the child, hoping for his recovery. The next morning, he had recovered fully, without any after-effects. His body temperature returned to normal, and his X-ray showed no inflammation. The boy was discharged from the hospital that day.

A child with severe brain paralysis also had a miraculous recovery with the help of hado power. A couple visited me with its baby and simply asked me to send my hado power to the boy. I shut out all thoughts from my mind and sent my power to him. Suddenly the parents exclaimed, "He moved his head! He moved his head!" They told me that doctors had said their son wouldn't be able to move any parts of his body for his entire life. After visiting me, they took their son to the hospital. The doctors said they had never seen anything like it, and that the son may soon be able to hold up his head on his own.

Animals and Healing

Hado healing is equally effective for animals. It can be even more effective because animals have such pure hearts and are sensitive to the healing power of hado.

I have two dogs at home, and both of them have been called "miracle dogs" by my neighbors and my veterinarian because of the way they recovered from illness. When one of my dogs was diagnosed with cancer, I wanted to heal him so badly that I held him to send him my hado power, even though he's the kind of dog who doesn't like to be touched very much. At first he resisted, but I think he understood what I was trying to do, so he became quiet and accepting. Finally, I fell asleep from exhaustion, while still sending hado to my dog. In the morning, my dog was still on my lap, and I felt that he was healed. I took him to the veterinarian, and the doctor confirmed that my dog's cancer had disappeared.

My other dog suffered from a serious liver problem. One day I took her to the same veterinarian for a checkup. Unfortunately, her liver problem was advanced and she needed to be hospitalized right away. I had a strong sense that she should be with me instead, so I took her home despite the veterinarian's advice. I prayed for her recovery whenever I had time. The following month, I took her to the veterinarian for another checkup. He told me that the blood test showed that her liver had started to function normally. He also said, "Frankly, I was surprised when you showed up with your dog. I didn't expect her to survive without hospitalization a month ago. Your dogs keep on surprising me. They are miracle dogs."

People often come to me for help in finding their missing cats. Just by listening to the client I can tell if the cat will be found or not. If I feel that the cat will be found or will come back home, I send hado into the cat, and the cat is always found.

Hado and Destiny

Hado cannot interfere with a person's destiny. I have learned this through my work as a healer. The following story is an illustration.

A client once called me about her sick father. "He has been diagnosed with terminal cancer and he is believed to be within six months of death," she said. "Can you do anything for him?"

I used my clairvoyant power to see her father. I had a vision of his stomach magnified in front of me, and I saw total blackness all over it.

"Is he suffering from stomach cancer?" I asked. She said he was.

I tried my power further and felt that I could heal his cancer. I told my client this.

"Is that true? Are you totally sure about that?" she asked.

"Yes; however, I think he will pass away for another reason. I see his fate," I said.

"Well, if you can ease his pain, please send your hado power directly into him as soon as possible."

I started to visit the client's father in the hospital once a week. Everything went well and he started to feel lighter and lighter. He was discharged from the hospital within six months, and I continued to visit him at his home. My client was so happy to see her father regaining his health.

Then I received sad news from my client. Her father had passed away. My client directed her anger at me and said I was a con artist who had cheated her and her father. I felt sympathy toward her because she had just lost her beloved father after having hoped that he might live longer; however, at the same time, I felt sure that I had healed the cancer.

A few weeks later, I received a letter from her lawyer. The woman was suing me for fraud. The letter also notified me that an autopsy was being conducted on her father's body. Another week passed; then the lawyer called to say that the woman had withdrawn her complaint. The autopsy revealed no tumors and concluded that the cause of death was a heart attack.

This story illustrates that when a person's time has come, hado power cannot heal the illness but it can help to ease the pain. No one can alter the fate of another person; it is out of our hands.

III

Messages from
the Dead

波動

I have recently begun to interact more often with people who do not understand Japanese. I often strongly feel that we can communicate without words but with our hearts. Strangely enough, after having conversed for a while through an interpreter, some people start to respond to me even before the interpreter opens her mouth. When I ask how they can understand me, they say that they just feel it in their heart. It looks as though hado surely works as telepathy, when people totally open their hearts.

The same thing happens when people receive messages from the dead. They have completely opened up their hearts to the dead and are willing to listen to them. Opening your heart to these messages can bring you comfort, lessen your pain, and help resolve any issues that may be lingering since the person departed from this world. Our souls go on living even after we die. Sometimes the dead want to rest in peace by fulfilling their hopes and delivering messages to the living; one way they communicate with people in this world is by releasing hado. Whether the messages are simple or profound, they are extremely valuable to those who are still living and want to keep the dead alive in their hearts.

Receiving Messages

To receive messages from the dead, the most important thing is your heart. You must have compassion, respect, and trust for the dead; then you can visualize them in front of you and tell them you are ready to receive the correct and accurate information. As a hado master, I often sense messages from the dead as a vision. Other times I hear their voices, and sometimes I even sense smells as if things were right in front of me.

Once, a client started to speak about her late father-in-law. Suddenly "tofu" came to my mind, so I asked her if she might know why. She looked surprised, then said, "My father-in-law really loved tofu, so I always had to prepare tofu, just for him, every day."

"I think your father-in-law is asking you to eat tofu for him sometimes. The next time you eat it, think of him and pray for the repose of his soul. He will be glad if you do that."

Sometimes the dead send messages with a smell. A businesswoman came to see me for help and took me to see her buildings.

"These buildings don't have enough tenants. Will you send your hado power to the buildings so that we will have good tenants move in?"

I started to send hado power into the building, but something unexpected happened. I said, "I smell kimchi [Korean pickles flavored with garlic] and fish. Do you know why?"

She looked surprised. "My grandparents were originally from Korea, and I constructed buildings with their estate. That must be the kimchi my grandmother made. She was from Pusan, a Korean port city, and they put fish in kimchi."

I kept sending hado power, and I had a vision of a fat, elderly woman with beautiful gray hair and a smile. According to my client, it must have been her grandmother. I guessed she was happy receiving the hado power.

After I finished sending hado into the building, my client asked me to send hado power into another building next to it. While sending hado power this time, I had a vision of an old man with a bald spot and a big smile. I asked her who it was.

"It must be my grandfather," she answered.

My client's grandparents must have had considerable feelings for the buildings because the buildings were built with their estate. Their thoughts and emotions were strongly connected with the buildings. In the end, my client's business did become successful, and good tenants occupied her buildings.

People who have passed away rarely speak. When they have messages for someone in this world, they usually show me a vision. I always ask my clients why I have these visions and for their interpretations.

Parents suffer greatly when a child dies, especially if the child's time comes when he or she is young. I would like to share two stories about dead children who gave me messages.

A mother who lost her son in an accident visited me. "I think my son wants to say something to me. Can you hear him?"

I told her I had a vision of a photo album and shoes. She replied, "I know . . . it is the photo album filled with the pictures of him taken at the summer festival."

This festival was something that he had looked forward to more than anything. The photo album filled with these memories was very precious to his parents. I felt that her dead son watched his parents delightedly when they looked through the photo album. At the mention of shoes, his mother said she still had regrets that she had forgotten to put his shoes in his casket. I told her, "I think I had the vision of shoes because you worry so much over them. Ask your son for permission to discard the shoes. I am sure he wouldn't mind."

The parents now enjoy the festival with their son's friends and invite them to their house. Even the smallest memory could be the most cherished thing for the family of a departed loved one.

An elderly couple who lost their daughter showed me her picture and said, "Our daughter was killed in an accident when she was only eighteen years old. Can you tell us how she feels about her short life? Because she died so young we feel that she might have wanted to do something before her death. If there is something she left behind, we'd like to do it for her so that she can rest in peace."

I sent my hado power into the dead daughter. Then I heard her saying, "Father, Mother, don't worry about me. My life was short but I did everything before I died. I did many good things and not-so-good things. I did everything that I wanted to do."

I explained what I heard to the parents. They started to cry and told me, "She said something just like that a few days before her death. Now we are sure that she lived her life to the fullest, with nothing left behind. Thank you very much." Their faces became very peaceful.

Some people are destined to have short lives; however, it doesn't mean that they don't live life to the fullest. Somehow, on some level, such people know that they won't live as long as other people do, and they accomplish what they have to do before their death.

Sometimes clients complain that they suffer from something that is cursed. In my experience, things do curse people, but it is rare. The following episode is one such rare case.

A friend asked for a consultation concerning her twenty-five-year-old nephew who lived on a tropical island. He was not sick or lazy but hadn't gotten out of bed for three months.

I sent hado power to the young man and had a vision of the neighboring landscape. I tried to visualize him in bed, and to my surprise, I saw a tail coming out from his hip. I kept sending hado power until the real figure was revealed: it was a turtle. I advised my friend to call her sister to check if they had a turtle in the house. There was, in fact, a stuffed turtle kept in a closet. I told her to take it out.

I sent hado power to the stuffed turtle, and after a brief interval, I saw a vision of the turtle returning to the ocean with joy. At the same time, the mother called me back with excitement.

"My son just got up from bed and started to wash his face. I looked at him in amazement, and he said, 'Mother, I am hungry. Can you cook something for me?' I served food and he ate everything with relish!"

I later heard that the son went back to a normal life thereafter.

I think that the turtle was not ordinary; he was exceptionally clever and had a special spirit. He suffered a lot when he died, and his last emotions and pains were left in this world and imprinted in his body. I don't think that it was the turtle's intention to harm the dutiful son, but he wanted desperately to go back to the ocean and had no choice but to ask the kindest person in the family for help.

I have found that stuffed animals have the strongest thoughts and feelings that can be left in our world and affect our lives. The effects vary depending on if they died in agony or died instantly without any pain. If they died in pain, their thoughts are left in our world and could be a curse. (I have found no problems with keeping seashells at home, however.) I hope that by reading this book you will develop your own hado power, have conversations with any formerly living animals in your home, and judge for yourself.

When the dead want the living to notice their pain and suffering, they may affect the health of their children or someone else connected to them. At such times, the most sensitive and kindest one in the family usually picks up the pain or the thoughts left in this world. The dead never mean to curse or haunt people; they just want the living to know their sufferings and possibly to remove them. And since the other world is a world of eternity, even if you remove the pain many years after their death, you still remove the pain eternally. You can often see this working when people in the other world are healed by the love of the living; the pain of the living will also be removed, or they will receive gifts in a mysterious way. The following stories are examples of this.

A single woman in her thirties called me and said in a sad voice that she felt that her body was heavy. I visited her home. During our conversation, she told me that her parents had passed away, and she showed me photographs of them. I started to send hado power into the two photographs in front of me, using both hands—my right hand for her mother, my left hand for her father. My right hand suddenly started shaking.

"Do you know why my right hand is shaking but not my left hand?" I asked her.

"Perhaps because my mother killed herself," she answered.

"Don't worry. I will send hado power into her so that she will feel all right."

A few minutes after sending my hado power, my hand stopped shaking. "Her pain is removed. Now she rests in peace," I told her.

After a little while, her expression started to shine. "Maybe it is just my imagination, but I feel that my body is much lighter."

After this, I continued sending hado power into the daughter and carefully observed her movements, which were becoming better and better. She had an easy carriage, as though she were dancing.

Another time, a widowed woman in her forties came to see me, complaining of terrible neck pain. Even doctors hadn't been able to help her. She also had a bad complexion. (In fact, it looked eerie.) I tried my clairvoyant power with hado and had a vision of a young woman who resembled the widow in front of me. She had been ill-treated by her mother-in-law, crawling on the floor and driven mad by pain.

"Do you have someone in your mind?" I asked the widow, after describing my vision.

"Yes, my neighbor told me a story about a woman who was ill-treated and killed by her mother-in-law generations ago. I hear that I look very much like the poor woman who was killed."

I sent hado energy into the dead young woman. I felt certain that she was haunting the widow who was like her reflection, wanting the widow to know her pain.

All of a sudden, the widow's face brightened and transformed into a peaceful expression. She said with a smile, "It's strange. My body feels lighter and the pain around my neck has diminished."

I told her that the pain of the dead woman had been removed. I also felt that the dead young woman enjoyed hot tea when she was alive, so I advised the widow to serve an extra tea for her when she herself has one and to pray for her peace.

Sometimes strong emotions of the living wander around like a ghost. Hado can be effective in forcing emotion from the living back to where it came from. A friend experienced this when she thought a ghost was haunting her daughter-in-law.

She said she felt a presence of something and that fumes from incense that she lit would follow her daughter-in-law throughout the house.

This seemed like strange behavior for a ghost, so I used my clairvoyant power to find out what it was. It was not a ghost; it was a strong emotion sent from a living person. I sent my hado power to the lump of emotion, commanding it to go back where it came from. My friend called me again and said that the fumes stopped following her daughter-in-law and dispersed normally. Later she told me that the lump of strong emotion might have been sent from the daughter-in-law's ex-husband. She guessed that he might have heard that his ex-wife had happily remarried and was jealous. When we feel strong emotions, we send that energy directly to others, whether we realize it or not.

I once visited an old married couple's house. After exchanging greetings, the husband showed me a picture of a woman. "She is my daughter," he said.

I immediately knew that she had been murdered. "Did she die an unnatural death?" I whispered to him, and he nodded silently.

The man asked, "Can you tell us what really happened to her?"

I started to have a vision of water—an ocean. "Did she drown?" I asked.

"Yes, my daughter's body was found at the seashore," he said.

"I don't know if I should say this . . . She was killed and the murderer hasn't been arrested. Is that right?"

The parents nodded with tears in their eyes, and asked, "Can you see who killed our daughter?"

I saw a man who pushed their daughter from a boat. It was the daughter's husband. I explained to them what I saw.

"I knew it," the father said. "After her death, my daughter appeared to me in a dream and said, 'Father, please listen to me. I was killed by my husband.' But I had no way to prove that she had really appeared in my dream. That's why I asked you to come see me," the father explained.

"He has to pay the price," I told the parents. "Your son-in-law will be swollen like a bullfrog and die."

He said, "He's already dead, Ms. Matsuzaki. If he were alive, I would do everything I could to have him arrested. Indeed, he died of pulmonary edema, with his lungs full of water."

If people die in a tragically—in an accident or by violence—their pain and sorrow are very strong and attach to the place where they died; therefore, you should never visit sites of accidents, tragedies, or war simply for fun or amusement. The strong emotions released there require peace and quietude. If you can't avoid visiting those places, pay your respects and never disturb the rest of those who perished there.

Before we depart this world, our dead relatives or loved ones gather to guide us to the next world. I saw this firsthand when a friend dropped by my house while her husband waited for her in the car. She visited me regularly, but that day she was with dozens of spirits, including one who looked European. I was overwhelmed and asked her, "Have any of your relatives lived in Europe?" She said yes but wondered why I saw many spirits. Later I heard that her husband had had a heart attack and passed away just thirty minutes after visiting my house. Those spirits were the guides who had come to make the husband's transition easier. After understanding this, I no longer fear death; when my time comes, I am sure that I will see my deceased son and father again, and they will be my guides to help in my transition.

I often feel the spirit of my son very close to me. I perceive his spirit as bubbles with very beautiful rainbow colors. I offer him a glass of beer at dinner when I feel his presence because he loved beer, and I can sense him complaining when I forget to do so. My son also loved to smoke, and I offer him a cigarette sometimes. When I feel my son's spirit near me, I light a cigarette and it stays lit; when I light one for him when I don't feel his presence, the cigarette goes out in no time. I think that he keeps busy even after his death, helping his friends here from the other world. But he is always with me when I need his assistance. When I visited the United States for the first time, he didn't come with me. I was accompanied by a friend, and he thought that I could make it without his help. When I visited New York for the second time in order to write this book, he accompanied me. He must know when it is important for him to be with me. He wanted to inspire me when I was working on the book, and he also wanted to see how his real gift to me turned out.

What Happens after Death

People ask me what happens when we die. I know from my experience as a hado master that the spirit goes to another world, leaving the last thoughts and emotions behind. Also I know that all the pain will be gone and that departed loved ones welcome us to another world. The manner of death doesn't matter—disease, accident, war, or even suicide—there is the same peace and rest in the end; therefore, death is not a bad thing at all, especially for one who is heartbroken and has huge sorrow and pain in this world. It is fortunate to pass away when the time has come. The longer we cling to this world, the more we suffer.

Further, the line between this world and the other is very thin; the dead become guardian angels who come to rescue loved ones whenever they need help. They are happy when we are happy and they share the sadness we feel and help us from the other world; however, I believe that babies, especially those who leave this world before starting to talk, go directly to God. I once visited a grave where a baby was buried, and I asked the baby where he was. I saw him sleeping peacefully with his thumb in his mouth, and he replied that he was with God. I asked several other questions, but he went back to heavenly sleep. I guess that those babies are so pure and innocent that they are free to rest without worrying about things on earth.

As a hado master, I have arrived at certain beliefs regarding the afterlife. I don't know if heaven exists, but I am sure that there's no hell. If there were a hell, why would we have fate or suffering in this world? The most important thing for us is to live our lives to the fullest. I am often asked about reincarnation. I think it is too painful for each spirit to repeat the fate and sorrow of this world. Previous lives are our ancestors, and future lives are our offspring.

I firmly believe that what we call "karma" exists. Whatever you have done to others will return to you somehow, whether good or bad. Considering the circulating nature of hado, it is easy to understand this concept. Once it's released, it will return to you. If you have bad karma but are lucky enough to escape it in your lifetime, it will come back to your offspring. If you did something very good but it didn't return to you while you were alive, your children or grandchildren will benefit from your good karma. If you tried very hard but you weren't successful, your children or grandchildren will receive the success you are due. Sometimes the songs of an artist become popular after his or her death, or a movie focusing on a dead person or a novel of a dead author becomes popular and everyone talks about it. Those artists may not have received all the rewards of their hard work during their lifetime, but their success lives on. If you are fully aware of the consequences of your conduct and behavior, you will realize how important it is to live your life to the fullest, regardless of success or failure, with a good heart and good intentions.

IV

How to Develop
Your Hado Power

波動

Everyone has hado power. When a child has a stomachache, the parents instinctively put their hands on the child's stomach and rub softly. They are using their hado power without realizing it. If your friends are feeling down, you hug them and lay your hands on their shoulders to cheer them up. You are unconsciously sending hado power to them. Hado power is that simple.

However, the output of hado power varies from person to person, as hado power is released through the physical body and every body is different. In my experience, skinny people tend to have a smaller output than larger people. People who are very active tend to release stronger hado. If you don't have an abundance of energy inside you, you cannot use it for someone else. If you have been told that you are a good chef or that you give great massages, there is a good chance that you have strong hado power. Hado power can be inherited. If you think that some of your family members have strong hado power, your chances of having it are very good.

If you find out that you have an abundance of hado power, please practice hado often and use it to benefit humanity. If you happen to have a small amount of hado power, you shouldn't be disappointed. We all can have different roles in this world, and each role is important. We all can have more than enough power to help ourselves and our loved ones through training. Love makes hado power far stronger. I have seen many examples firsthand of people developing their hado power with practice and using it to improve their lives and the lives of their loved ones. The most important thing is to practice it every day, and you will feel your energy grow.

Although everyone has hado power, you have to be born with a special facility to reach a master's level. Everyone can play basketball, but only those with a special talent for it can become professional basketball players. To become a hado master, first you have to be healthy, both physically and psychologically. Second, you must have strong ethical and moral standards, because if you use hado in the wrong way, not only will you hurt others but you will also hurt yourself or your loved ones, due to the circulating nature of hado. Hado masters are generally at least middle-aged because you need life experiences in order to be compassionate and understand others' emotions.

As you begin to practice your hado power, there are a few things to keep in mind. In previous chapters, I described in detail how I perceive and send hado power; however, the way of feeling and using hado power is different in every individual, just as everyone has a different face. Please develop your own way through practice and training. You may find that you are stronger in some areas of hado than in others. For example, my son was good at pointing out where people or things were; that is not my strength, although I can describe what they feel. Discover your strengths through your practice.

If you are sick or feel weak, please regain your health before you practice or use hado power, because it requires a lot of energy and vitality. When healing a loved one with hado, first seek out a doctor to check your loved one's condition, especially if he or she is suffering from a serious disease.

Never use hado power for negative purposes. Some people try to practice hado power by bending spoons, for example, but I don't recommend that hado power be used for any destructive purpose, even to the least degree. If you are tempted to use hado power for destruction, remember that hado circulates, and it will return to you sooner or later. Even if you can escape it in this lifetime, it will return to your children and grandchildren.

Sometimes hado works in ways that are unexpected or beyond human understanding. It tends to reveal secrets and things that are hidden right in front of people's eyes; therefore, even if you try to use your hado power for criminal acts, the chances are that the authorities will find out about it in some way. Several times after I cleaned houses with hado power, the couples living there end up finding out about a secret love affair in a strange way, or an old lie comes to light that leads to the couple's separation or even divorce. Mother Nature first tends to reveal the true figure of a problem deep inside; otherwise, it cannot go to the root of the problem.

Hado power can do almost anything. Here is a partial list of the abilities you may be able to develop through practicing the lessons that follow.

- Distinguish between good and bad
- Manipulate the essence of materials (such as changing the taste of food and water)
- Understand the meanings of signs
- Help to heal diseases (physically and psychologically)
- Find people's (especially children's) hidden talents
- See the past and the future

- Receive messages from the dead
- Remove people's (both living and dead) agony and pain

Lessons to Develop Your Hado Power

Remember that the most important thing is to practice hado every day. You may also want to look at my picture or have this book close to you while you practice so that you can be connected to my hado power. Let's get started.

1. Feel the *Hado*

Lesson A: Nurture your sensitivity to hado by trying to feel the difference in the heaviness of the air when you are outside your house and when you are inside. Even in a small room, the density of air varies; usually the air in the corner is heavier than that in the rest of the room. Try to feel the hado in a room by scooping up the air in both hands. Then move to another room and scoop up the air again. You can feel the weight of the air and understand the difference.

After enough practice, you will start to feel the difference in the air. For instance, when you are walking down the street, you will start to sense which houses are releasing warm and comfortable hado and which are not, without knowing who is living there. When you are at home, you may start to feel the best hado spot in your house. (Usually that spot is already taken by your pets.)

Lesson B: Listen to music. Some singers have hado power and imprint their hado energy into their songs. This is why some songs linger in your heart, even though the singer may not have a great voice or technique. See if you get a stronger sense of hado from certain singers or songs.

Lesson C: Visit a museum. You may find that some paintings or sculptures have stronger and lighter hado than others. If it is good hado, try to receive the energy. If you go to a museum with ancient relics or tombs, you may be overwhelmed by the pressing hado in the building. If you feel that it is overwhelming, block yourself from the bad hado by saying, "Bad hado cannot come near me," or use another method that works for you.

Lesson D: Send your hado to a painting or photograph. After sending enough hado, you will be surprised to find that the colors become more vivid and embossed—the art literally becomes three-dimensional. (In fact, some artists ask me to send my hado power into their works before they enter contests.)

Lesson E: If you love to watch sports, you can practice your hado power by watching competitions. For beginners, practice with one-on-one sports, such as boxing. Before the competition, compare the density of the air released from both players and guess which one will win. (You don't have to be there in person; the hado can be felt from a distance.)

2: Change the Essence of a Material Object

Lesson A: Pour a small amount of water into a glass. Drink it and remember the taste. Hold the glass for at least a few minutes while visualizing me. Drink the water from the glass again. See if there is a difference; if not, dump it out and pour new water into the glass. Repeat the same process until you taste a difference.

Lesson B: Cut an apple in two. Put one half in the refrigerator. Take the other half to another room and send your hado power into it. Imagine the movement of the air in the room. Aim at one small point on the surface of the apple half, move the air into it, imagine the exit point, and release the air from there. Do this exercise for at least five minutes. Finally, eat the apple half from the refrigerator, and then the half you sent hado power into. Taste the difference.

Lesson C: Place two flowers in separate areas of a room. Look at one flower more often than the other. Only give attention to that one and send your hado power into it. Think strongly that it will stay healthier and live longer. You will find that the flower you give attention to stays alive longer than the other.

3: Learn Healing Techniques

After successfully changing the taste of water or apples, start learning healing techniques. (Of course, you can start with this lesson right away if someone in your family is sick.) If you want to exercise your hado on someone else's body, it is important to have permission from that person, especially when you need to touch him or her. It is also always a good idea to open the windows and the screens in the room before practicing so that the bad hado energy released from the sick finds exits.

Lesson A: Rub the affected area of your loved one softly with your hands. While rubbing, try to visualize me so you can be connected to my hado. Rub until the sick person feels warmer and lighter.

Lesson B: Make exits for the hado by pressing parts of the body. If you want to send hado power into an arm, press the elbow, fingers, and palm carefully. If you send it into the legs, press the bottom of the foot; for the head, neck, or shoulders, press the top of the head, temples, and back of the neck. You don't have to press hard; you just need to stimulate the area softly. Finally, imagine the movement of air; try to feel the snowflake-like particles of hado circulating inside the room. Aim at one small spot near the affected area and move the hado directly into the spot. Imagine that the hado circulates inside the body and is released from the exits you made. Practice this for as long as you can stay focused.

When you send hado power into someone's body, his or her stomach may start to make noises, or the person may start to feel warmer.

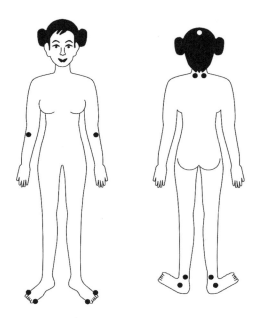

These are good signs that your hado power is getting stronger.

Lesson C: If you want to send your hado power to someone who lives away from you, just think of that person. He or she will receive your hado power. If you want to send it more effectively, visualize me, then close your eyes and feel the person in front of you. Let's say that the person has a problem with his or her heart. Visualize the shape of the heart magnified in front of you and send your hado directly into the affected areas using your fingers as an antenna for hado power.

Lesson D: If you want to try self-healing by using your own hado power, here's something you can try: First, pour warm water into the bathtub. Then send the hado power into the water by visualizing me and white snowflake-like particles. Soak in the tub and enjoy the warm water filled with hado power. You also can try techniques from lessons B and C in this section to heal yourself. In such cases, try to relax the entire time.

Additional Hado Lessons

Change the Taste of Food

1. When you cook, cook with love and wish that the food turns out delicious and that everyone enjoys the meal. Take note of how the food tastes. Then the next time you cook the same food, try thinking of someone you dislike or an incident that made you upset. Can you taste a difference between the two dishes? (Refrain

from practicing this exercise often, as cooking with hatred is not good in the long run.)

2. When you make bread, hope for the bread to be delicious and visualize me. Compare the taste to bread you do not give this attention to.

3. Place two bottles of beer in the refrigerator. From a distance, send hado very carefully into only one bottle. When you feel enough hado was sent into one bottle, open the bottles. Before you taste the bottle you didn't send hado to, visualize hado being removed from the bottle, just in case it received hado by mistake. Taste the difference.

Self-Healing Techniques

1. Visualize in front of you the part of you that's suffering and send hado to that area. For example, if you are suffering from an ulcer, you may see some parts of your stomach that are darker; send hado power into those dark parts. (It is more effective to practice this technique when you are soaking in the bathtub because your cells are more supple when you are in warm water.)

2. Visualize your body in front of you. Then apply pressure to the top of your head to make an exit. Visualize the air moving into your feet and then moving up toward your head. When you do this

exercise, you may feel that your body becomes warmer as the blood circulates better inside your body.

Healing Techniques

1. Visualize in front of you the sick part of the person you want to heal. Then visualize that same part on your body, just to make a comparison. In my case, if the patient is suffering from an ulcer, I see the troubled parts dark; if the patient is suffering from cancer, I see the cancerous parts white. You may see it differently. Send hado power into the sick part.

2. Take a piece of paper and a pen. Draw two people. (The drawing can be very simple.) Imagine that one is you and the other is the person you want to heal. Then put your hand over the drawings and feel the difference between them. You may feel that the sick person is heavier, or you may feel the sickness in a different way. If you become more advanced, you may start to feel that some specific part is heavier than other parts. After feeling the difference, send hado into the drawing of the patient, hoping for his or her recovery. When you send the hado, send it from the feet or legs to the hands or head.

Other Occasions

1. When someone is suffering from misfortune, visualize that person and send hado from the feet toward the hands or head. You may want to use the scooping technique I described earlier. The scooping technique is originally used to feel the difference in the air, but it is also useful to send hado to someone.

2. If you want to send hado power to your pets, you can send hado from the bottom up to their head, as if you are scooping the air. If you do this directly, apply pressure to the head to create an exit before sending hado power.

In any exercises, don't try to accomplish the goal in one day. Do the exercise every day, little by little. This is the key to make your hado power strong.

Believe in Miracles— You Can Do It, Too!

As I say repeatedly, hado power comes from your heart. Just by thinking of or caring for someone, you release your hado power to that person, and it can make a difference. Can you imagine how much you could accomplish after developing your own hado power?

I do believe in miracles; I believe that I can make a difference in people's lives with my hado power. I usually pray for their recovery or happiness while I'm sending my hado; however, when I have very difficult cases, I block all thoughts from my mind, as if I'm practicing Zen meditation. I devote myself to it because people can do things beyond their normal ability when they shut out idle thoughts from their mind. You can even perform miracles with this technique.

Nothing is stronger than love. If I can make miracles, you can make miracles for your loved ones, too.

V

Tips for Living Healthier and Happier with Hado Power

波動

Stagnant Air at Home

Is your ventilation system at home working properly? It is very important that air in closed spaces has mobility and finds exits; otherwise it starts to release bad hado. For example, hotels with many guests have light and good hado because the continuous opening and shutting of doors makes the air circulate continuously.

I have seen many clients whose houses are filled with stagnant air. They hardly recognize it because they get used to living in that environment. One client told me, "My father has been suffering from autoimmune disease for a long time. Maybe because he has been staying home all day, he has become weak, and lately he has started to complain about chest pain. Now he is in the hospital. Will you send your hado power into him? It is painful to see him suffer for so long."

I used my clairvoyant power to see her father and sensed that the problem was coming from his house.

"I think I have to visit his house; otherwise, my hado will not be fully effective in this case," I told the client.

When she took me to his house, I was overwhelmed by the dark and hazy air inside. I told her, "Please open up all the windows and exchange the air *now*!" After the stagnant air was dispelled, I started to send my hado power into the house.

The father was in the hospital at the time and had no idea what was happening in his house; however, he recognized that he didn't feel any chest pain or nausea at the same moment that the change in his house occurred. In fact, another patient told him that he had a much better color in his face that day. Also, the shadow that had been observed on his chest X-ray disappeared after I sent hado power to his house several times. The doctor discharged him from the hospital in no time.

Clean the air in your house. Open all the windows, screens, and doors and exchange the stagnant air for air filled with good hado from Mother Nature. Using the scooping technique I introduced in chapter 4, find out which rooms have heavier air. Then try to circulate the air in those rooms, especially the heavy air, toward the window. (It is a good idea to use a fan.) Move the air in the upper corners of the rooms with extra care because that is where bad hado usually lingers.

Receive Good *Hado* from Mother Nature

The easiest way to receive good hado is to visit nature: walk in the forest, camp alongside a pure stream, and go to the beach. This pure hado stays with you only temporarily, so you should connect with nature as often as you can. One day I met a friend who was releasing exceptionally beautiful and powerful hado energy, which made me want to stay with her for a long time. She told me that she had just gotten back from the beach. I have felt the same type of strong hado from Hawaii; when I visited, my lower back pain vanished, and I almost forgot about it. As the airplane approached Japan on my return, the pain came back to me. No wonder people want to go to these special places on their vacations and older people want to live there after retirement!

If you live in the city and have no time to visit nature, or if you want to receive good hado all the time, try to have lots of plants in your home. Without exception, plants release good hado; the bigger the trunk of the plant, the stronger the hado it releases. If you are planning to renovate your house in the near future, it is a good idea to use wood flooring because wood releases comfortable and strong hado energy. If possible, choose a thick flooring; the thicker the wood, the stronger the hado.

Do not expect flowers to release hado energy that will cleanse your house. Flowers use all their hado power to bloom, so they are something to enjoy purely for their beauty.

Make Your Jewelry Shine

Jewelry touches your body directly and tends to absorb your negative energy. With the help of plants, you can cleanse your jewelry, too. First, open the windows and screens; then put your jewelry near the base of strong plants and leave it there for a while. If your jewelry has absorbed a large amount of negative energy, you may want to leave it there all day. Also, you'll see a difference if you put the jewelry near the window and expose it to the air and sunlight on a dry, sunny day. After the jewelry is cleansed, you will be surprised at how shiny and light it becomes.

Clear Out Negative Possessions

After absorbing human thoughts and emotions, inanimate objects start to have their own energy. Sometimes they release bad hado in a home without the occupants even realizing it.

I received a call from a client who complained that there was something amiss in her house. Her son had nightmares every night, and he said there was something eerie in his room. I felt that the air was condensed in the upper corner of her son's room. I asked my client if there was something there, but she told me she couldn't recall anything. I told her that I would visit her house.

Entering his room, I carefully inspected the corner. As I had expected, there was something hanging on the wall—a small mask from overseas. The face on the mask looked very sad and depressed. I asked her, "Where did you get this? Did you bargain over the price when you bought it?"

She told me that she had bought the mask on a tropical island and had asked the artist for a discount. I told her, "I think the poor artist spent all day making this mask with all his heart, hoping to make ends meet; however, you bargained for it and he couldn't get enough money to support his family. His heart is imprinted in this mask."

Then I started to send my hado power into it, hoping to ease his disappointment. After a while, the face on the mask became peaceful. After this, her son was able to sleep deeply, although his mother never told him what had happened.

Go through your house and take stock. Be aware of any feelings you detect and any object that gives off vibrations, especially if it had a previous owner. Try removing the object from your house for a time to see if that has any effect. If the hado in your house improves, get rid of such objects permanently.

Choose Your Living Space Carefully

Previous owners' thoughts and emotions are imprinted in dwellings. Sometimes residual feelings are so strong that they control subsequent occupants' feelings and behaviors. I am sure that what we call "haunted houses" exist; in such houses, the emotions of dead people are imprinted so deeply that even people who are not sensitive to hado energy can feel it. I have also experienced houses where good and cheerful feelings of the previous owners were imprinted.

Be careful the next time you hunt for an apartment or a house. If you have already moved into a new place and you feel bad hado inside it, I recommend that you exchange the air as often as you can, especially by moving the air in the corners. Buy strong plants with thick trunks and put them where you feel the bad hado stagnating. If those methods are not very successful, you may want to think about moving because your physical and psychological health are most important.

If you cannot move, you may want to try the following method: Choose a sunny day to cleanse your house. First, prepare salt water; open all the windows, screens, and doors; and turn on air conditioners and fans, if you have them. Ask everyone to leave and to stay out until the procedure is finished. Pour the salt water onto the ground around the building, asking the salt to purify it. While you do this, try to picture me. Finally, visualize the air inside each room moving to the exits, such as windows and doors, and leaving the building. Repeat this visualization until all the air exits. Don't get close to the building for at least ten minutes because you don't want to expose yourself to the dense, negative hado energy that is leaving.

Understand the Laws of Nature

Even if you receive plenty of good hado, you cannot benefit from it if you have bad intentions.

I used to imprint my hado power onto blank empty cassette tapes or CDs and give them to my clients when I felt that they needed some extra help. I told them to play the tape whenever they had time so that they could receive my hado power directly whenever they needed it. When the tape or CD broke, I told them to throw it away because its life was over and it had released all my hado power in exchange for receiving negative energy. When cancer patients used my tapes, they reported that the tape became like ashes when it was torn. (I wondered whether tumors also became almost like ashes in their bodies.)

One day I gave a tape to a young male client. He called me and reported that his tape was torn in a short period of time. As I knew that he was a very healthy man, I asked him what he had thought of or wished for when the tape was torn. He told me that he asked the tape not to get caught by the police when he was street racing with his friends! I guess that even the tape felt bad by hearing his wish.

Appreciate Your Guardian Angels

People ask me if everyone has a guardian angel. Japanese people believe that close relatives (usually parents or grandparents) who have departed are your guardian angels; therefore, indeed everybody has guardian angels. They protect you no matter where you are, no matter who you are. You don't have to do anything special for your guardian angels, but it is good idea to show your appreciation whenever you feel you've been protected or whenever you are happy. When your guardian angels are happy, you may feel a chill, as if the room temperature has dropped.

Look for Meaning in Signs

It is always good to think about the meaning when things break or disappear in a strange way; it could be a sign of what is to come. Before a change or an important event, you are often shown a sign. If you nurture sensitivity to hado, you will start to understand the hidden messages in your everyday life. A sign can be good or bad. If you think that a sign is bad, pray and ask your guardian angels to protect you. If you think that a sign is good, show your appreciation to God and the guardian angels. If things break on your behalf, thank them for their sacrifice.

Have Sympathy for Others

When you see an ambulance or hear sad news on TV, feel sympathy toward those who suffer. As I say repeatedly, hado is sent to others simply by thinking of or feeling sympathy for them. If a thousand people pray for the same thing with good will, the power of the prayer is magnified. When more people start to understand the power of hado and use it properly, they can make miracles happen.

Coping with Difficulties

From my experience as a hado master, I've learned that each of us has a fate. After a long, hard day, you may feel happy, and the amount of hardship decreases proportionally. Or you may suffer because you are about to bring something important into this world; this could be considered a kind of labor pain, and you cannot quit until you finish it. Before God or Mother Nature, human beings are equally small. Little tricks you may try have nothing to do with your fate. Accept your fate and wait until the storm is over, because everything has an end, sooner or later.

Time moves on, although people cannot always see this. Please don't give up hope, because you cannot know when you will receive good news; you may even hear it tomorrow.

It is not a good idea to move or change your job when you are feeling unfortunate. Good and bad fortune go around in a circle, just like the changes of the seasons. You may be in the winter of your life right now, waiting for a warm spring—you don't want to wander around in a heavy snowstorm. Keep a low profile and wait until a better time comes. Patience is the key to coping with difficulties.

When you feel that you can no longer bear the hardship, ask God or your guardian angels for help and tell them that you have suffered enough.

If you have lost something very important, think of it as a sign of a turning point. Be prepared for a significant change in your life.

Never be envious of someone else's good luck. Never say bad things about anyone else. If you need to let out your anger, do it in a positive way. When you think about someone, hado will be released from you to that person instantly. Never do anything with bad intentions. If you happen to release bad hado, you don't want it to return to you. In some cases it comes back to your loved ones, and you don't want them to suffer from your malicious intentions.

Hado resonates with similar hado. If you have negative hado, you will attract negative hado, too. Keep your spirits high and be positive whenever you can, and positive hado will come to you.

Finally, I have imprinted my hado power in this book. Whenever you feel that you need my help, please read this book again. You will be connected to me, and you will find your way after receiving my hado power.

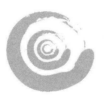

Appendix

The Hado Support Group Handbook

After reading this book, you may want to tap into your own hado power. You may find it helpful to form a support group because group exercise is sometimes a more effective or easier way to draw forth your potential power. When you see someone in your group successfully change the taste of water, you will think, "Well, if my friend can do it, I can do it, too!" This feeling removes the barrier of your underlying skepticism (which unintentionally blocks your heart) and helps develop your own hidden ability.

The following material can assist you in organizing your own support group.

1. The purpose of the support group is for each member to develop his or her own hado power by assisting one another.

2. Agree on when to start and how long the meeting should last. Most people's concentration lasts one to two hours at a maximum. If you are a beginner, it is enough to practice for thirty minutes. Notify another member if you will be late or cannot attend a meeting.

3. Rotate the meeting site. Before the meeting, open doors and windows and turn on the ventilation system to exchange the air inside.

4. Participants should read through this book before joining a hado support group in order to understand the concept and the nature of hado power. Start your training by referring to chapter 4, "How to Develop Your Hado Power." Do not hesitate to modify the lessons in the book. The most important thing is to continue the training in the most comfortable and convenient way.

5. As you advance, discuss and compare your perceptions and experiences of hado. Remember that everyone senses hado differently and there is no correct or incorrect way. Through discussion, discover your strengths and weaknesses.

6. Discuss any signs that you see. Discuss what the signs might be trying to tell you.

7. Honor the confidentiality of personal matters discussed during meetings.

Important Reminders

- Never use hado power for negative purposes, even to a small degree.

- If you are not in good condition or feel sick, take time off. Get your strength back first, as using hado power requires a lot of vital energy.
- When you try your healing technique with other people, it is important that they visit a doctor and check their condition before the practice.
- Open doors, windows, and screens when you try any healing techniques.

There are no hard-and-fast rules for developing your hado power. Please relax and enjoy your practice.

If you discover anything through training that you would like to share, please write to me:

Toyoko Matsuzaki
c/o Beyond Words Publishing
20827 N.W. Cornell Road, Suite 500
Hillsboro, OR 97124-9808
or send feedback through my Web site,
www.hadopower.com.

Information on upcoming seminars will be posted on my Web site, and also on my publisher's Web site, www.beyondword.com.

Message from the Author

When you are sick or feel pain in your body,
Put your hand on the affected area and
Visualize me.
You will get better.

When you need to change your life,
Or feel that you will never find a glimmer
of hope,
Visualize me.
You will find a way.

You may realize the difference right away,
Or you may need to wait a bit to feel it,
But the change starts as soon as you read
this book.

You may find it unbelievable,
But you can lessen your burden
By getting to know me.

I have imprinted my hado power into this book.
It will give you the power
To make your life better.

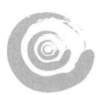

The Healing Power
of Hado CD

In support of *The Healing Power of Hado*, we are very pleased to offer three unique CDs from hado master Toyoko Matsuzaki. These special CDs have been imprinted with Toyoko's strong hado power. Hado is a life-force energy known to have healing powers. The benefits of hado energy are purified air, a balance of your body and mind's energy level, and positive changes in your health, relationships, and work.

By simply playing the CDs, you will experience Toyoko's hado power remotely. This hado energy cannot be copied from one CD to another. Only the original CD from Beyond Words Publishing has been imprinted with this special hado power. The length of time CD's can release good hado depends on the environment. If you find that your CD breaks or does not play after some time, this means that the CD has released all of its good hado into you and your environment and absorbed as much negative hado as it can hold. In this case, please discard the CD and replace it with a new one.

Choose from the following three CDs according to your preferences or situation.

Water of Hado

This CD's sound is produced by the purest water running from a spring deep in the forest in Nara Prefecture, Japan. This CD is ideal for relaxation or meditation. It is also perfect for offices and shops as background music. The hado power from this CD will purify the air in your environment. As a result, you may experience an increase in business or sales.

Music of Hado (Oboe)

Oboe played by Ryusuke Yoneyama, professor at Wakayama University, Japan

Great for music lovers. This CD is ideal as background music for homes, offices, and shops. The hado power from this CD will purify the air wherever it is played. When the hado power is released in your home it cleanses the air to contribute to your good health. It can also help relax children and help them get to sleep. In the workplace, the result is a more balanced energy that leads to an environment more conducive to business. As a result, you will attract the right people and see an increase in sales.

Silence of Hado

This CD is designed specifically with **NO MUSIC OR SOUND**. Although it is silent, the hado power will stream into the room while it is playing. This CD is ideal for those times when you don't want to be distracted by sound for example, while sleeping, driving, meditating, studying, or working). It is also an excellent aid for those who are ill or recuperating from an illness. The young are especially receptive to hado energy; play the CD in the nursery and your child will experience a longer, uninterrupted slumber.

Produced and directed by Toyoko Matsuzaki
Recording Engineer: Yasuo Yoneyama
Duration: 30 minutes (approx.) each

Calligraphy (Heart & Abundance)

Hado master Toyoko Matsuzaki designed and calligraphed each letter with great care. She also stamped it with her official stamp. Each autographed design of "Heart" and "Abundance" releases strong hado power. This power may be used to absorb the negative energy in a room or to maintain balance. These beautiful characters emanate hado while purifying the air in the room. They balance the energy level of your body and mind, thus improving relationships and attracting the right people. As they are all hand-written, each letter varies slightly. Perfect as gifts or for home decoration.

Other Books from
Beyond Words Publishing, Inc.

The Hidden Messages in Water
Author: Masaru Emoto
$16.95, softcover

Imagine if water could absorb feelings and emotions or be transformed by thoughts. Imagine if we could photograph the structure of water at the moment of freezing and from the image "read" a message about the water that is relevant to our own health and well-being on the planet. Imagine if we could show the direct consequences of destructive thoughts or, alternately, the thoughts of love and appreciation. *The Hidden Messages in Water* introduces readers to the revolutionary work of Japanese scientist Masaru Emoto, who discovered that molecules of water are affected by thoughts, words, and feelings. Dr. Emoto shares his realizations from his years of research and explains the profound implications on the healing of water, mankind, and earth.

The Power of Appreciation
The Key to a Vibrant Life
Authors: Noelle C. Nelson, Ph.D., and
Jeannine Lemare Calaba, Psy.D.
$14.95, softcover

Research confirms that when people feel appreciation, good things happen to their minds, hearts, and bodies. But appreciation is much more than a feel-good mantra. It is an actual force, an energy that can be harnessed and used to transform our daily life—relationships, work, health and aging, finances, crises, and more. *The Power of Appreciation* will open your eyes to the fabulous rewards of conscious, proactive appreciation.

Based on a five-step approach to developing an appreciative mind-set, this handbook for living healthier and happier also includes tips for overcoming resistance and roadblocks, research supporting the positive effects of appreciation, and guidelines for creating an Appreciators Group.

Come to Your Senses
Demystifying the Mind-Body Connection
Stanley Block M.D., with Carolyn Bryant Block
$14.95

Come to Your Senses: Demystifying the Mind-Body Connection teaches the reader groundbreaking techniques that will change your life forever. The book offers the reader how to find and demystify your Identity System (I-System) a key component which controls your mind, body, and soul. It is a powerful way of achieving a happier and healthier way of life within days.

Water Crystal Oracle
Based on the work of Masaru Emoto, author of
The Hidden Messages in Water
48 Water Crystal Cards, $ 16.95

Masaru Emoto, author of the best-selling book *The Hidden Messages in Water*, discovered that molecules of water can be affected by our thoughts, words, and feelings. When water is frozen, the crystals reveal the concentrated thoughts directed toward them. Included in Water Crystal Oracle are 48 beautiful water-crystal images to both enhance your life and balance your well-being in many ways.

Ocean Oracle

What Seashells Reveal about Our True Nature
Author: Michelle Hanson
$26.95, boxed set (softcover with card deck)

Combining the ancient art of divination with the mysticism of seashells and their interaction with humankind throughout time, *Ocean Oracle: What Seashells Reveal about Our True Nature* borrows from many disciplines to produce a new and inspiring divination system based on seashells. The boxed set is comprised of 200 full-color seashell cards, a companion book, and a four-color foldout sheet with overview plates of the 200 shells. Appreciation for the shells' aesthetic beauty is enhanced by the text descriptions detailing the animals' behaviors, abilities, interactions with humankind, and their meaning. The shells serve as tools to assist you in revealing subconscious, hidden beliefs and attitudes.

To order or to request a catalog, contact

Beyond Words Publishing, Inc.
20827 N.W. Cornell Road, Suite 500
Hillsboro, OR 97124-9808
503-531-8700

You can also visit our Web site at *www.beyondword.com.*

Beyond Words Publishing, Inc.

OUR CORPORATE MISSION
Inspire to Integrity

OUR DECLARED VALUES
We give to all of life as life has given us.
We honor all relationships.
Trust and stewardship are integral to fulfilling dreams.
Collaboration is essential to create miracles.
Creativity and aesthetics nourish the soul.
Unlimited thinking is fundamental.
Living your passion is vital.
Joy and humor open our hearts to growth.
It is important to remind ourselves of love.